GW01048673

A
TROUBLESOME
DISORDER

BEING AN ACCOUNT OF AN INTERVIEW WITH MASTER FRANCIS BARBER, SERVANT OF THE LATE DOCTOR SAMUEL JOHNSON

DAVE RANDLE

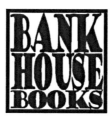

A TROUBLESOME DISORDER

First published 2002

ISBN 1-904408-00-1

© 2002 Dave Randle

Published by BANK HOUSE BOOKS

Printed and bound by
Lightning Source UK Limited

Designed and typeset in England by
BANK HOUSE BOOKS
PO Box 3
NEW ROMNEY
TN29 9WJ.

FOREWORD
by
G.W. Nicholls, PhD, FRSA
Erstwhile Curator of the
Samuel Johnson Birthplace Museum

In this novel, Dave Randle reconstructs a meeting in Lichfield in 1793 between an unnamed reporter and Francis Barber, the negro manservant of Doctor Samuel Johnson. Johnson had died in London nine years earlier and Barber had brought his wife and children to live in his famous master's home town. The novel follows their conversation, principally about Johnson, as they walk around Lichfield or share their meals together on a single day. The reporter comes to understand the range of Barber's intelligence and his confused feelings for Johnson, and in doing so begins to appreciate something of the nature of slavery and freedom.

Francis (or Frank) Barber had been born in Jamaica and was brought to England as a little boy by a friend of Johnson's. About the time of his wife's death Johnson took Frank into his house where he fullfilled the roles of servant, companion, and surrogate son to Johnson. He was educated by Johnson who also oversaw his religious and intellectual development. In his youth Barber fled from Johnson's service on several occasions, most notably when he ran away to sea. He was only discharged from the navy when Johnson contacted acquaintances in the government. Barber accompanied Johnson on several of his trips around the country. He later married a white woman and had several children, and for some time they all lived under Johnson's roof. On Johnson's death in 1784 Barber inherited most of his master's fortune. On removing to Lichfield however he proved unable to manage his finances and he and his wife fell upon hard times. Frank died in Stafford Infirmary in 1801.

Randle's novel combines close research with imaginative and sensitive speculation. It deals at once with a peripheral life, lived out as an appendage of a great man, and also lets us understand what it meant to be in such a situation. It explores the feelings of an intelligent and kindly treated negro in Georgian England. In doing so the novel makes a statement about slavery of different kinds and the difficulties of living with freedom.

GENTLEMAN'S MAGAZINE - 1793

AN EXCURSION FROM WALTON TO LONDON

Contributed by our ingenious Meteorological Journalist, who, being at Lichfield upon the 21st. of June, after visiting the Cathedral, where he attended the morning service:

Sent for Mr. Francis Barber, 35 years the humble companion of the late Dr. Johnson, who, with his family, now resides at Lichfield.

Francis is about 48, low of stature, marked with the small-pox; has lost his teeth; appears aged and infirm, clean and neat, but his cloaths the worse for wear; a green coat, his late Master's cloaths, all worn out.

He spends his time in fishing, cultivating a few potatoes, and a little reading.

He laments that he has lost the countenance and table of Miss S—, Mr.— and many other respectable good friends, through his own imprudence and low connexions.

He was the companion of Johnson, for, as Master, he required very small attention. Francis brought and took away his plate at table, and purchased the provisions for the same. But if Francis offered to buckle the shoe, &c., "No, Francis; time enough yet. When I can do it no longer, then you may."

He was his companion in the evening, when the domestics made a circle around the fire, when the Doctor chatted and dictated. "Why do you not ask me questions?" the Doctor said to Francis.

"But I never could take the same liberty with my Master as with another person."

The companion in his journeys, and at Streatham, when Francis preferred Streatham; but, when London had more attractions, he returned to London, and left his Master at Streatham.

"You never heard your Master swear?"

'No. The worst word he ever uttered, when in a passion, was: 'You dunghill dog'."

The Doctor would never suffer himself to be denied, which often put him to inconvenience when busy, on which occasions, he either wrote in the night, or retired into the country.

Mr. Barber appears modest and humble, but to have associated with company superior to his rank in life. The benevolence of Dr. Johnson appears strong in his treatment of his servant during his life, and in his liberal bequest to him at last.

It seems it was out of his power to render himself very useful as a servant, yet the Doctor would not cast him off on that account. And when the Master was no more, he provided a staff to support him in his stead.

Besides, Francis is oppressed with a troublesome disorder.

I had to regret that my short stay would not admit of longer conversation.

CHAPTER ONE

IN WHICH YOUR REPORTER GOES ABROAD IN LICHFIELD, ATTENDS A SERVICE AND COMMISSIONS AN ERRAND

All notions of ease or slumber are early put to flight in our modern coaching inns; The Swan being no exception. This fact is the more true on the Sabbath, when, to the general clamour of the Inn's own comings and goings must be added the plaintive pealing of the church-bells and the bustling of their answering congregations.

Though unpleasing, to be sure, such untimely commencement of the day went not so ill with your correspondent one June morn in the year of one-thousand-seven-hundred-and-ninety-three as it otherwise might, his travels allowing of but that day in which to discover and interview a most particular subject.

Even at that early hour, it was something warmer than would allow much comfort to those appropriately drest for the Lord's Day, and the wispy, insubstantial clouds presaged the likely pattern of it. Having the scientific appellation, *cirrus* (the which proceeding from their wool-like character), these last are now recognized by those learned in the science of meteorology (among which your correspondent makes bold to claim place) as sure evidence of a succession of balmy and settled times.

Travelling, as is my unvarying practice, with certain instruments for the determination of such matters, I was further able to ascertain, (ere I quit my chamber), that an excess of that air-borne moisture, styled, humidity, would render the local atmosphere oppressive to a degree. Being one of few persons thereabouts skilled in the aforenamed science and, thusly, better enabled to prosecute the cause of his own comfort, your correspondent clearly perceived the advantage of seeking out cooler interiors and putting himself to no avoidable exertion; resolving, accordingly, to have his subject brought, in preference to troubling his own person upon the dusty thoroughfares of the town, when the sun would be at its most fiery.

Having broken my fast with some good country fare - and put into a better humour by it, you may be sure - I made my way (in what I believe to have been cloaths of exactly the right sort - neither too rustick, nor yet too fashionable, but suggestive of quality and sobriety) to the lowest gallery, or boardwalk, hallooing as loud as may be, amid the constant commotion, for anyone who would earn a penny.

Whether my cries were lost in the general noise, or that indolence and unwillingness to shift commonly to be met with in people of the lower sort disinterested them in my generosity, it was some little time before any one could be induced to come forward. He that did was, methinks, a child of one of the grooms; small and stocky, his speech of the most barbarous sort, so that even a prodigious traveller, such as your correspondent, found great difficulty in making it out.

After much business, he was off upon his errand, and I had liberty to go abroad in the town, with the object of attending the service in the cool of the Minster, while the boy could search out the subject of my article for *The Gentleman's Magazine.*

I had been several times privileged to enjoy the company of that great Englishman, Doctor Samuel Johnson, while he yet graced the World, so was soon able to discern among the better—quality inhabitants of his native town, that manner of speech, or accent, whose melodious tones and soft edges often took the sting from his sharper utterances, making them much the less offensive in the life than in the writing down.

It was, indeed, in some connexion with the Doctor that I had placed this visit to Lichfield upon the itinerary of my tour of the midlands, the details, if you will grant me your patience, becoming clear as the account of that singular day unfolds.

The mail-coach for Wall being, for a reason I could not immediately ascertain, stalled in the through-way, I quitted the inn-yard by edging through the shadow beside it, taking great care, as you can be sure, that it shouldn't set off before I could gain the street.

My arrival having been under cover of darkness, and the coach-flaps closed against the night breeze, I had taken little impression of my surroundings. I now realised that a second coaching inn existed on the opposite side of the street. At the moment, the *Pleasaunce* was newly arrived from Stafford and must needs take up the whole carriageway, including the side of the road adjacent to the Swan, in order to make the turn into the George, with the result that attendants, waiters, and other employees of the Swan felt themselves under an obligation to bawl abusive oaths and unflattering descriptions at all servants and patrons of the George, particularly the ostlers, engaged at that time upon guiding the leading horses, while letting fly with their feet and sticks at the curs snapping at their heels.

With a final rumble, the bigger coach achieved the entrance and I stood my ground as the four mail horses felt the whip and, digging yet another ditch with their hooves in the already well rutted surface, by degrees, got the coach and its complement of frightened passengers into dusty motion; at which, the curs, briefly cowed by the blows of the ostlers, seeing now a new quarry, fell again to their yapping and snapping, at the heels of the horses, and the wheels of the coach, until someone therein throw them a morsel or some bones upon the high road.

You may be sure, my kerchief fast to my face, I allowed a goodly time for the dust thus created to settle, which, doing so, discovered not merely that section of the London to Stafford Road called Bird-street, but my first glimpse of a part of the Minster: the extreme tip of one of the three famed spires, its light-coloured stone in sharp relief before the purest-blue sky.

Bird-street was all motion. A little way off was yet a third ostlery, at the sign of the King's Head, being the staging post for Roodsley and Birmingham, which confirming your correspondent's intuition that the greater part of the population of this market town is now engaged upon the servicing of the travelling publick, its employment and its quartering all included within an hundred or so paces of this outskirt.

The first street after Bird-street is still the Market-street, with close courts and alleyways, and troublesome vendors and beggars seeming to have the concerted object of discountenancing the visitor. When oaths (and the meaningful brandishing of a cudgel) can disperse this tiresome rabble, a person mayhap to find the liberty to gaze upon the house in which the great dictionary-compiler drew first breath, and lived out his early life.

Though it be solid, and of good character, there is naught of the grand about it, leading others to liken it to the good Doctor himself. The roof is a little high-crowned, but the windows are of generous size, giving the whole a not displeasing aspect; being a description not at all to be applied to the personage who deigned to answer the street door thereof, at the expense of many knockings and pummellings. This apparition must be concluded to be some antiquated female relative of the present habitant - its sex to be deduced more from its apparel than its hideous visage and unwigged bald pate. No cajoling could prevail upon the apparition to stand aside, any more than to offer intelligible communication. Being unwilling to protract such demented intercourse, I cannot now report on what might have come of the interior, and must regret that I have never crossed that historical thresh-hold.

Before the house was a pleasant gathering of bread-sellers, some of which most comely, as they saunter to gain the custom of those of all stations; and what a world of bread! Upon their heads, sometimes steadyed by a slender arm, sometimes balanced by a sweet comportment, are trays of golden buns; or cross-woven loaves; bread-rolls, crusty pyes and loaves of all other sort: white-floured, stove-bread and 'Thatch-Cottage'.

The towne of Lichfield supports many bakers, the cereal being grown by the crofters hereabout and the milling by the windmill on the mount beyond the Minster. There are also two water-mills, though one having been lately closed by the work of landscaping undertaken on the Minster Pond, the other being at the drain of Stowe-Water or Pool.

You may be sure that the fresh-bak'd bread made a pleasant effect upon the senses, much to be desired in lieu of that proceeding from the 'sun-bak'd' kennel in the market-place close by.

It being the Sabbath, none but the bread-hawkers and some

flower-sellers were installed that day, but the congestion was none-the-less considerable, for the cobble-stoned market-place is a mean affair, encroach'd upon by both a minor chapel and the Church of St Mary.

This edifice, with its stout tower, was the regular place of worship of the Johnson Family, the cleric therefrom having performed the office of Young Sam's baptism - though 'twere not done in the church, there being doubts concerning the sickly child's survival and, accordingly, the pastor being summoned to his birth-chamber in the house opposite. The Family Pew was here, though we are informed that the Doctor did not often occupy it, having been many years 'in the wilderness' as the Church would have it. A short time in this refuge from the hot streets may be spent in contemplation and thanksgiving for that one, who not blest by his Maker in the physical way, nor by birth, yet took his place among the Great Men who are the envy of the lesser nations.

Repose finds no place in the life of the hard-prest journalist, and I must needs reach the Minster in good time for the Service, for I was desireous to see the memorial lately placed there by the people of Lichfield to their celebrated son.

My path took me from the Market-place to the Conduit, taking its name from the funnel or leat, ingeniously constructed in olden times to carry water from the Damme to the bakeryes, all water having been previously fetched from the Bore-Well, which was much guarded by the monks.

The continuation of The Conduit is called Damme Street and has some shoppes for trinkets, crosses, chandels, incense, votives and other stuff of a religious connexion. Likewise confections are offered to entice the faithful back to the paths of Indulgence while yet their devotions and repentance are in their ears!

The Damme is an object of antiquity which, though fashioned by hand from stone and mortar, has been reclaimed by Nature, tuffets of grass and small trees thriving in the cracks of its venerable parapets and providing fine perches for the multitudes of birds - pritty swallowes and jet-black corbyns being the greater part of their number.

On the west side of the Damme is the Minster Pool, as it is now to be known, though it had been a cisterne formed from the meeting of some brookes, of which the main being the Lemon, called simply Damme Pond or Mere. The late transformations of the 'Swan of Lichfield' — the poetic Miss Anna Seward — require for it a title more descriptive and romantick.

That the poetess has improved upon Nature, your humble correspondent would not venture to doubt; that the act of poetising at this place may cause a 'want of poetry' further downstream is not to be thought upon. The Yeomen, crofters, millers and fishers will make shift, as they ever have done, to amend their lives in respect to the poetic vision, you may be sure.

Naught much more than a trickle escap'd the eastern side of the damme on that summer day which, passing by the silenced mill building, went down to the Stowe-pool, some way below. This water is given by Nature majesty and form in measure superior to that of the other pool, notwithstanding its 'improvements'. Separated from the messuages and dwelling-houses of the town, it appears at once, clean, tranquille and unspoilt. The only buildings near it are tumble—down manufactories, ivy-clad and nettle-thronged, taking nothing from the beauty of the whole.

That entry to the south-gate of the Minster Yard should be made as difficult as may be by the beggars which foregather there, you will not be surprized to read. These fellows and their doxyes would put even the London beggary to shame with their clutching, pulling and wheedling, and their whining refusals to accept the Lord's Judgement. Ever too open in my dealings with humanity, I credited overmuch the idiots' capacity for reason, taking pains to put forth the proper explanation of the incorruptibility of the journalist and his ethical obligation to abstain from affecting (whether for good or ill) those things it is his duty to disinterestedly describe.

As you, Dear Reader, will readily understand, this is no easy precept to live by, usually requireing great resolution and fortitude (I will not add: strength of character), but it availed me naught with these wretches, and I had no course but to lay about them, it going against my Principle, but bringing no appreciable or lasting change to the pattern, of their lives, while enabling me to gain the Close without further delay.

The Minster has, at various times in its long history, been a fine ecclesiastical building, though I found it wanting some attentions. Those renovations that went forward in the early part of our present century may now be discern'd only in the ledger-books. A general sense of neglect now pervades the structure, both in-side and out, and there seems little willingness or regard toward it from the local people or the clergy either.

Indeed, there was a plan afoot, not long since, to sell off all the treasures and valuables, even including the lead from off the roof, th'ungodly having so far taken the precedence! Our good Johnson busied himself in putting an end to that particular folly.

And here, now, is his memorial — not ostentatious — to be found in the South Transept, adjacent to his childhood friend, Garrick. The more affecting for its simplicity and personal warmth, it bears this inscription:

"The friends of SAMUEL JOHNSON, LL.D. A Native of Lichfield, Erected this Monument, As a tribute of respect To the Memory of a man of extensive learning, A distinguished moral writer, and a sincere Christian. He died Dec. 13, 1784, aged 75."

The service was well enough done, the quire being most practised, and giving, in that worthy cathedral, an harmonic resonaunce the equal of any to be heard in my long travels. Indeed, this hardened reporter must own to a tear or two in the *Te Deum Laudamus.*

An accommodating native identified the more notable of our fellow-worshippers: here were Levetts, Giffords, Furnivals, Cranleighs, Wrights, and there was our landscaping poetess who, my guide ungentlemanly informed me, the "swanliness"having "gone to roost", is known now among the common—people as the *"Turkey* of Lichfield"!

Leave-taking done, I took the quick way across the Close,

13

lest my Subject be arrived at the Inn.. and growing impatient. By this fashion is it possible to come out into Bacon Street, crossing what has been a bridge back into Bird Street, the Swan upon the right hand.

Gaining the welcome cool-ness of the saloon, I hastened to the booth or parleur to which I had directed my Subject be brought. The young whelp with whom I had charged his delivery attempted to importune me at the entrance door for the other half-penny of his hire, so I must perforce advise him that I would first be satisfied with the conclusion of his part ere I could consider the service full rendered.

Not without some trepidation, you may be sure, I grasped the brim of my hat and circled the 'high-backed settle whereon my curious Subject attended my arrival.

CHAPTER TWO

IN WHICH WE MEET MASTER FRANCIS BARBER AND LEARN
SOMETHING OF HIS EARLY LIFE IN THE SERVICE OF DOCTOR
JOHNSON

Mr. Francis Barber is a Negro, native of Jamaica, and, for thirty-five years, the humble companion of Doctor Samuel Johnson, as well as being his residuary legatee, which should find him in good comfort here and accustomed to some ease and elevation among the provincials.

But the figure who rose now and returned my bow exhibited no luxury of dress or evidence of being well-used by Life. Though his years should be but forty-eight (as near as he, himself can reckon, his birth obscure), he appears aged and infirm. He is low of stature and wore, upon this occasion, a green coat, his presentation clean and neat, but his cloaths the worse for wear and all ill-fitting, being his late Master's cloaths, all worn out.

His voice was broken and raucous, and his manner of speech, though cultured and of good address, bearing the marks of old-age and dis-ease, so that he says: "Franthith Barber, at your thervith", which peculiarity resulting from the loss of his teeth.

He removed to Lichfield about a year after the death of his master, the affairs having then been settled, with his wife, Elizabeth Barber, a white woman, to whom he has been married these seventeen years, and lives now in a house in Stow—Street, where he spends his time in fishing, cultivating of a few potatoes and a little reading: this he informs me while we get at our ease, I calling for some of that Lichfield Olde Ale whose fame was propagated by Mr. George Farquhar in his *Beaux Stratagem*, a prelude to good conversation and dinner.

Just as his years could not account for his look of age, so it was immediate strange that he seemed to grow younger with animation and with ale. A light rekindled in his black eyes, and his movements grew looser, though he became bowed and slow again while he lamented his current life.

He appeared, I ventured, to have had two distinct lives: one of great interest and stimulation, in the company of his marvellous master; the other, his present retreat from the world of wit and fashion; the former being but a dream from which he must now be rudely awakened.

He returned that any such retirement was not of his desireing, low connexions and imprudence having denied him the associations with Quality he valued as the highest prize in his legacy, and begg'd leave to amend my categorisation of the parts of his existence: "For I have had *many* lives," quoth he, "Nor do I doubt that I will have more, ere this world will have done with Francis Barber."

His words were singular of themselves, but something in the manner of their delivery conveyed a deeper import which could not be receiv'd, e'en by a person as experienced in the ways of the world as the present writer, without an involuntary shiver.

Returning to myself, I regarded him coolly for some moments, using the device of sampling the Swan's fine ale to regain my advantage of him, but nothing in his bearing or in his person suggested aught of mirth or jest. I deemed he was in earnest. His gaze was steady, though oft-times he seemed to be regarding something not present; not, that is, visible to any but he.

My time was short, and I was anxious to get from him all I might, so, selecting my words with care, I re—opened the interview: "Per hasard, if I have not got the full measure on't, I may still report that spent with Doctor Johnson was one of your lives; your current existence another?"

His answer was ready: "If so, of which of those lives are you part?"

My wit, which had little exercise since quitting London, was warming now: "I visit you in the second in the cause of the first." I was not displeased with this riposte, but, again he was ready:

"Then you belong to that which you call my first life, and I am happy to call 'first among my lives'; and, although, like Mister Garrick, you find me engaged upon a new Play, it is still my 'servant' you would have news of."

My interest was quickened by this, withal that I am not accustomed to being made sport of by those of a lower station.

"'Tis not a pretty way of repaying hospitality, sir, to endeavour to best your host, but I'm a match for't and will go along in the service of that inquiry after knowledge which is my animating principle."

His eyes had been far off, but returned. There was even the hint of a smile on his gummy mouth. "Take no offence, I beg you. As you have accepted, I was long in the company of a man to whom niceties ran a poor second to the witty construction, and, as we move from life to life, we are wont to take some mementoes with us. That quickness and intelligence which was the joy of my lamented master lately excluded me forever from the company of Miss S— and others of her circle.

"Thus did what I brought with me in the way of custom and comportment from my life in Jamaica make me unfit company for Colonel Bathurst's household."

I bethought now that I began to see how he compartment-ized his life in a number relating to the major reverses of direction therein. A simple matter, then, demanding no further enquiry, so I ordered the wench to have food set before us and fell to my original purpose of interviewing him upon the finer details of his life with Johnson.

I bade him give me a full description of his duties as servant, these being in no wise clear from the chronickles of his master's life.

"Be assured," he returned in a way which spoke again of a strength or power greater than his appearance would suggest, "that he of whom you speak had more lives even than I, in many of which I was of little or no significance, which is why my doings are not recorded; but, in others, I played a greater part, there being, at times, none present but he and I, which is why our doings *cannot* be recorded."

Twas plain to me that this was another pretty trick, by which he would make himself more interesting and protract the hospitality, but he took another liberal swallow of beer and continued:

"My publick duties were not too many. It was my practice to answer the street door to callers, and to give whatever attentions were required to the master's person, these last being so few as to be almost without existence until he came to be ill near the end. My other duty was the table, for which I bought the provisions, (the grosseries from Mister Sancho who, good in the way of trade, was also a cultivated African, like myself), took. charge of the preparation of, and waited with upon my master and such guests as there were. I also performed this office at places where my master and I would visit; such places as Streatham Park."

His eyes moistened at this, and he took some more ale. "Nobody will ever begin to comprehend how much I miss him."

Something of this poor black man's plight caused my sympathyes to well up, and, for a few moments I took his hand (in a companionable and manly way, you may be sure), and felt me honoured to be privy to his private grief.

The soup arrived now, and I made shift to lighten the air: "It would have been part of your duty, though, to see to the Doctor's habit, and lay out his cloaths, I don't doubt?"

A successful ploy, this, since his humour so much, and so swiftly, improuved as to turn to laughter!:

"It would surely be to my eternal mortification if any aspect of Doctor Johnson's physical presentation were lay'd at my door. I'd think that a valet who sent his master into the world, a—purpose, as *he* was wont to go would be deserving of the gallows! Do you be serious, Master Reporter!"

There seemed, once more, to be a mysterious change in him as he laughed. He was strange to behold, his hot black eyes narrowed by mirth, and his mouth revealing his pink gums, yet it was not possible to gainsay his joy. The laughter fell from him, as it had been waiting to be released, and, at its end, he seemed less bowed—down, less ancient, less used—up.

He arranged his napkin (most acceptably) and prepared to do such justice to the pottage as a man with no teeth may. I saw that he regarded me once more from deep within his eyes: "I thank you, sir. It is long indeed since I had cause for such levity. It can not be valued too highly."

In an endeavour to maintain his good humour, and lead him to speak further of his late master, I begged leave to suggest that he must have known happiness in periods of his life.

"That I have, sir," he replied airily, while soaking a wad of oat—bread in the soup, "as may be easily deduced from the fact that I have lately known great misery. He that has not known happiness, though he live his life in want and suffering, stands not at a sufficient distance from his misery to know it as such, believing his condition to be the norm. That expansion of the senses wrought in me since being taken from my native land has given me great capacity for pleasure, to be sure, but it has made the reverses, though the depths of which appear luxurious to the common-folk, the more difficult to support.

"You wish to hear that I was happy in my late master's household, and 'twas often so. Yet, there is another face to the coin and, as I had not then experienced real misery, so I failed to place the full value upon my fortune, indulging often in resentments and jalousyes, and holding off from the experience of pleasure for fear of pain.

"By the time we have sufficient education to fit us for a life, that life is done, and we must enter upon another."

I had not thought to hear such sentiments, or such philosophizing from a servant, and found it did not sit easy with me, tho' I think I continued to give a good appearance of *sang-froid* to my guest. Merely the insistent assurance, to myself, that this person was a singularity, enabled me to hold on to the sense of order which, if his insight and mental powers were commonplace among his class, would surely and irremediably break down.I recalled that the Doctor had expended much upon his companions' schooling: "You would appear to have profited much from your own education. Doctor Johnson must have been well-pleased in you."

"My school-life occupied close on six years, taken in two parts, albeit more than twenty years between them. I'm sure that is as long a period of teaching as many can boast.

"I have little recollection now of the time spent at the Reverend Mister Jackson's school in Yorkshire — the place was called Barton. I was yet a small child, new arrived from the Carribee, and all seemed passing strange. The people there were simple and direct, with no affectation, and I was not ill—treated. The schooling was very elementary in the academic way, but I learned to like order and neatness, both in deed and in thought; a capital lesson for an existence such as mine is.

"My life there ended with that of the Colonel Bathurst; it, like myself having been his property.

"I clearly recall the mixture of elation and terror I felt when Doctor Bathurst" (the Colonel's son) "told me about the Will, when I was come back to Lincoln.

"Suddenly, I was a freed man — a state for which I had no fitness or preparedness — and I had been left twelve pounds, which was more money than I could ever imagine. Thus do values alter by the store we place upon them. I should have gone into the Cathedral and given thanks, but it frightened me. The tower wheeled above my head. My senses were all disordered by these unlooked for changes, so that I ran away, and kept on running until I am come to the River Meadow, the Cathedral and the House now safely small and far off.

"I looked into the water and recalled how, two years before, my Jamaican life had finished. All my sisters and brothers there as if they never had been. The boy that worked and play'd with them was gone from them. I was not alive in that existence, and now my life at school, and as the Colonel's kept-slave was finished.

"Francis the slave was dead and gone, and to be thought upon no more. This new Francis must make his own way. He was his own man; no master to guide him, but himself.

"A great weight had been taken from me, but it was as an anchor from a ship. I realised I would be adrift in uncharted waters, so resolved to offer my services to that same household from which I had been freed, until I had sufficient of age and knowledge to try the world."

"In which you demonstrated precocious wisdom." I could

readily see how his resolution to inter forever parts of his life that had been painful, or were otherwise cut off from him, had been of great service in his bearing with his frequent vicissitudes, and was pleased to determine that it was a simple device, not needing further investigation, which, none the less, I complimented him upon.

"Simple device? Say you so? Well, perhaps that is how it began, for the import of it was truly not seen by me at that time. Indeed, many veils then remained to be lifted, and the time for their lifting still many years off. Looking now at that life from this great distance, I cannot easily isolate the moment of death, or of rebirth."

I began to find his mystifications tiresome. "If I remember aright, you came soon into Doctor Johnson's household."

"I had met him on a number of previous occasions, in the company of Doctor Richard (Bathurst), and reverenced him from the first.

"We shared a difficulty of going unnoticed which, I believe, drew us, one to the other. He acknowledged me always, in a fashion to which I was, by no means, habituated. He would inquire about my education, consult my poor knowledge, and seek to know my opinion on this or that part of his beloved London. My opinion had mattered to no one before, and I had not expected that it ever would."

"You had visited London, then?"

"I had *removed* to London, since that is where Doctor Richard lived. He could not really afford my service, but took me with him to London after his father's death, that my education and preparation for the world might be expedited.

"It was thus that I came to accompany him to Bromley for the interment of Mrs. Johnson, when it was put forward that Doctor Johnson might be in need of a companion in his grief. He was not for it at first, I believe, but was inconsolable in his loss, and Doctor Richard was concerned that he might pine and waste him-self, if there were none to see to him. His only company was then the Williams woman who, even allowing for her afflictions, was far from being a consolation. What she lacked in eyesight, she better than made up for in tongue. I could never abide her."

"Yet, did she not live at your master's various houses for most of his years in London?"I asked him, finding it difficult to accept that she was such a disconsolation to Johnson in that case.

"Aye, sir. The devil whose creature she was kept her a-plaguing of the rest of us as long as may be. My master, for his part, was a better Christian than 1, for he suffered any one, no matter how undeserving, to receive succour, if it was his to give — often, indeed, when it was not, he having borrowed or begg'd more than once for no comfort of his own. He treated Mrs. Williams, at all times, with great respect, dining in her company, and bringing honoured guests into her presence, as if she were a Royal Personage.

"I believe this to have been another example of that contrariety of character which also led him to his kindnesses to myself. He had always the principle of doing the opposing thing to that expected of him — and 'twas not another of your 'simple devices', for his care and respect, once so whimsically directed, was never other than honourable and genuine, for all that it could appear mischievous to some other.

"He was soon led to relent in my regard, and I removed to Gough Square a little over a week after the laying to rest of Mrs. J. The house was very well-placed, being no great distance from the commerce of Fleet Street, nor from the printers with which he must deal in the preparation of his Dictionary. Also he would never suffer himself to be denied, so could easily reach the inns and taverns from here; Charing Cross, likewise."

He said this last with a peculiar leer, so that my sense of delicacy and respect for the departed precluded further inquiry, though bringing certain thoughts, all unbidden, to my mind.

'Twas timely, therefore, that the wench should arrive with the spitted larkes. They had taken long enough to be sure, but I had called for them to be particular well-done upon observing my guest's want of dentition.

Of a sudden, that person took a different course, announcing:

"You must know, sir, that I had not the ambition of remaining perpetually in service."

I did not know this, and had always assumed that there had been no other, certainly no preferable, course, his faithfulness to his master being the leading principle in all authoritative literary allusions to him.

"No, sir, I had received in the will of the colonel a thing too valuable to be lightly set aside.

"Just as happiness is to misery, so those born into freedom, wot little of it. And, had I not been allowed my freedom, I should not have been discontented to dedicate myself to the service of such a one as I was now called to.

"But the colonel's will must be answered, and I must guard my rights thereunder. I would not be cowed or brought to servility without I stood upon my own recognition. I would not receive the orders of the Williams woman, and would take time of my own for my own purpose.

"Doctor Johnson had a quick comprehension of this, and never demanded meniality, but the household accorded me no respect, it having multiplied with the years, and I soon came to possess sufficient of age and intelligence to seek the greater world.

"Also, if I may say so, my amorous propensityes were strong, and early developed. Curiosity brought me many conquests among women of all sorts, and I was, by no means, ill-favoured for their satisfaction."

What manner of talk was *this* from a guest at table! What a fellow I was to dine with! Still, I fancied I might have a notion as to the reason for his premature physical decrepitude!

Following this confidence, his eyes became once more fixed upon his inner thoughts, and we ate for some moments together in silence, he volunteering nothing further, and I content to muse upon what he had so far said.

The larkes having been done justice, he pushed the plate from him and, grasping the pot of ale, lolled back from the table in an easy and familiar fashion. "You can speak of a man being free," he said at last, "but, if he have neither income nor property he hath no freedom in the *world.*

"When I deem'd myself ready to quit the house in Gough Square upon that first occasion, I went forth with such as was remaining of the Colonel's money and chose my own paths. Believing myself master of my own time, I chose this moment to sleep, that to rise, this other to be at a place of my own choosing, these many to be spent in pleasurable pursuits and company.

"But it soon came out that I was master of nothing. I had not knowledge nor property enough to hold out against the forces of the world.

"Long, indeed, did it take me to see that, of such knowledge and property as I had, the former was and remained the Doctor's, and the latter was and remained the Colonel's. Though passed to me, I had none of it.

"Brought low, then, and too ashamed to return to the house, I must find a position to live, and lay aside all pride.

"While I had still a little for food, and could hold my person respectable, I was admitted to the service of Mister Farren, the apothecary, from the recommendation of Doctor Levet, who was the best of those in the house (My master excepted) and was my friend. He walked, each day, great distances to minister to the common people who had no money for medicaments and doctoring in the ordinary way, but he had learned his skills in Paris from some famous chirurgeons there, and would use them for the benefit of the poor, which was not liked, and he was called 'strange' for it.

"He came to Mister Farren for his concoctions end brought me news of Gough Square and my master. I think now he reassured him of me, though he feigned to keep my secret. He was a greater friend than I had wit to recognize.

"He afterward married to a woman that he used to meet in a coal-shed in Fetter Lane; he believing her to be a good woman, and she thinking a doctor must be well-to-do, they were both surpriz'd and the marriage ruined, which I was sorry for.

"At Mister Farren's, I studied to learn something to my advantage, and came to know a little of physick, which I have had cause to value, though I could wish I had not. Th'apothecaryes of Lichfield have lately taken from me more than ever I could have gotten from Mister Farren, my eldest daughter being now in a constant affliction."

His look suggested that he had regretted this last remark, it being unhappily close to home, and he sensible of the unworthyness of complaint. He resumed his narrative with some haste:

"But physick and concoctions is only drugging; a man's humour not repaired by it, only a phantasm laid over. It is well enough to put a face on it, when there is no other thing than suffering. My friend Doctor Levet eased the suffering of many. A worthier man never lived. "'His useful care was ever nigh', my master wrote. It is no longer, and there is none to replace him.

"When he told me, so that I could believe it, that Doctor Johnson missed me, and would have me back, if I would come, with no inquisition, I was moved in my heart, and could not rest until I had gone to him, though I had not served notice to the apothecary. Mr. Farren was a good man and very comprehending and I believe Doctor Levet spoke for me.

"A convivial and joyous lachrymosity attended our reunion, which was not the case with Mrs. Williams, but I was so happy from being returned to Doctor Johnson, that I did not permit her to sully my humour, but simply hid her blind-stick and smiled the more at her redoubled curses and profanityes.

The boiled mutton was now come with some good summer-vegetables. I had formed the opinion that Master Barber gave good enough value, so ordered some Port-wine to accompany it, the ale, excellent though it was, something heavy for the main course.

Mistress Anna Williams had known some popularity as a poetess, but it was naturally to be supposed that the affliction of blindness had altered her character. "So, was Miss Williams accustomed to use immoderate language in the house?" I asked of him.

"I think you may say that. Her vocabulary was, in every sense, remarkable; the more for one claiming gentility and having literary pretension. The flash-talkers by the Hummums should be hard put to it to best her. The Doctor was passing tolerant of her, making nothing of her tantrums, ever declining to respond in like kind."

"You never heard your master swear?"

"No. The worst word he ever uttered when in a passion was: 'You dunghill dog!'" He smiled anew at this. "I will not tell you to whom he was referring."

Laughing now companionably, we felt a little easier one with the other, and I gave him no pressure to continue, while we made something of the mutton, with the assistaunce of the entirely (and unexpectedly) tolerable Port.

CHAPTER THREE

IN WHICH MASTER BARBER TELLS US OF HIS LIFE AT SEA AND FAVOURS THE PATRONS OF THE SWAN INN WITH A CHANTEE

The midday sun had now gone over, its amber rays slanting through the low window of the saloon making a patch of light and warmth on the flags near our table and an overfed-looking feline coming, flopped it down in the midst thereof.

Seeing this, Master Barber, taking up the side-dish that had held the pease, placed of his mutton in it and lay'd it before the creature.

"Thou art free with the provender, I see, though I believe you to be without affluence yourself."

"Yes, sir. I never see a cat wanting, and share such as I have with them. I owe a debt to their kind, for, in the world beneath the house in Gough Square, only the Doctor's cat, Hodge, was worse used than I; he being roughly appriz'd of my returning discontentment, when there was none other to tell; he alone being un-fitted, if not un-minded, to peach to the master!"

"You did not easily settle back in your old home, then, I conclude."

"You conclude well. I think it was something of my progression to full adult-hood, more so than any real change in the household, for my master's house was never much for order or repose and, though it differ'd from all other, it seldom vary'd of itself. But I was beset with sullen humours. My master rarely quit the dictionary attic, except to go abroad, for he was busy upon his *Idler* and his *Rasselas*, and I could no-wise tolerate the other in-mates. I was often put in great distemper by matters of small import, and came, at last, to be disgusted by the flirtations and dalliances there play'd out.

"For what reason, I knew not, nor sought to discover, but that I tried with all my will to impose order where there was none; to make those things of which I did not approve cease to be. So forcefully, indeed, did I exert my mental powers upon the projection of such an effect upon my surroundings that I brought myself to a compleat stand-still, my will, occasioning no exterior compliaunce, returning upon myself.

"This served to defeat my anger, but drove me into intense pity for my condition. I could not utter a word but I would be disposed to weep. It was as I should have a lump in my very throat, so I desir'd no food, and kept my bed for days together. My master came and asked what ail'd me, but I could say naught, whereat he pray'd by my bed, telling me the value he plac'd upon me, but I could not accept it, and even dis-liked him for it; may I be forgiven. He bade Doctor Levet concoct something for my throat, but I cast it away, and my distemper returned, so that I poured scorn on all present and wished them d—d, quitting the house, all at once, and presenting myself at the *Recruitment* with the passion still upon me.

"My resolution did not falter, and I was soon enroll'd upon the frigate ship, HMS *Stag*, as a land-man, under the command of Captain Tindall."

"What impulse led you to the nautical life? 'Twas surely the last course Doctor Johnson would have wish'd for you, his opinions on the matter being well-known."

"As to that, sir, there was an element in it of being what none other would wish me. I was free to assert my independent will only in what was contrary to the will of others. Though what they wished for me might be all to the good, I had no part in it, which I saw still as a form of slavery. For good or ill, I had need to make mine own decisions, what-ever outcome being of mine own cause.

"I believe that my young mind also made some association between liberty and the sea. My homeland of Jamaica is an island, reliant upon the ocean for all things. I was born with the smell of the salt, the mewing of the gulls, and the creaking and flapping of the sailing ships already within me, and part of me.

"No freedom may be dream'd of in that land, that does not entail crossing the ocean; not a poor Jamaican who does not dream of a better life beyond the horizon, whether in the promise of England, or the memory of Africa. My earliest recollections are of hiding in a tree-top, watching the white ships come and go. From my perch, they were not big straining things full of sugar and people; just beauteous objects, suggestive of a world beyond. Only when I was taken away, riding with the Massa Colonel in his phaeton, did I meet with the sailors; seeing them sing and dance and play their whistles. They were strong men with a hard life, but they were not bowed down, and they knew much of the world. They must take orders, but kept up their spirit of defyaunce, so that they were never slaves."

At this, he regarded, with some pointedness, his empty goblet, which, in replenyshing, I smiled, in-wardly thinking: to be sure, this Master Barber has little of the slave about him!

"My livery made them respect me, so that they told me tales and were quite taken up with me, which helped me turn from the faces of my brothers and sisters whom I could not easily bear to leave. Also, I made fast friends with the cabin boy, who taught me many games and tricks, and the tyeing of knots. But he was a slave like me, because some of the sailors made him do things which brought him in great shame, so that he could not speak of them to any soul but me, and would never again be free, though he return one day to his family, for he could not own his life.

"It is likely that his words were part of the influence in my putting to sea, for they remain with me now as at the moment of their utterance:

"'If a man be not master of his own person, he can be done with hope and fear, for all is as one to a being with no soul, which is what a slave is, his master having possess'd of him, and taken the precedence'.

"It was his first voyage. He told me he had resolved to jump-ship when we reached Liverpool, but I never heard of him more; though I have often thought on him, hoping that he managed to make good his escape, and was able to make him a new life."

"And what of you? Found you life 'before the maste', as the saying is, agreeable?"

"That I did, sir, I'm bound to say, for that we were all doughty men together, with a common task, and that it was a life of companionable-ness the like of which I had never known."

At which, he gave myself and the others in the saloon of the Swan great surprise in coming of a sudden to his feet and commencing, in his broken voice to perform a *chantee*, elaborating the same with such salutings, gyrations, gestures and muggings, as seem'd to defy his arthritick frame:

> *"For it's ho! me mates and hi' me mates,*
> *"Wherever we may roam.*
> *"Though we're out for war, or we swarm ashore,*
> *"Still the sea shall be our home.*
>
> *"And it's haul the ropes, and wind the ropes;*
> *"To set the sails or ride.*
> *"This bully crew be strong and true*
> *"Which cannot be deny'd!"*

You will readily imagine with what merriment the revellers and diners in that place greeted th'outlandish sight of this small black man (he, something of a figure in this place) displaying such anticks and giving out how the "Thea thall be our home"! Many were the bangings on the tables and the *"bravos"*ere we could resume our conversing, and the land-lord, entering into the spirit of the thing, and grateful that the communal jollity would improuve his commerce, bade us drink each a measure of Jamaica rhum 'upon the House', Master Barber saluting of him and downing the same in a single swallowe. I acknowledgeing his kindness, but regarding the acid-seeming liquour with more circumspection."

The King's Navy was busy in many parts of the world in the middle of the century, with campaigns in Canada, engagements in the Americas, difficulties in India; and the interminable nuisaunce of the French had not yet entered the period of quietude pursuant to the Treaty of Paris. "You give good account of yourself as a matelot. To what distant corners of the world did your career take you, and upon what adventures?" I was keen to know.

"The furthest reaches of our voyages were Cromarty in Scotchland, where the enemy was the cold, and Tor Bay, where the enemy was the cyder, which caus'd several of the landing-party to fall over the boards."

"What? So you were never out of friendly waters?"

"No, sir, for the Stag was upon the business of fisherye-protection; preventing the foreign fishers from poaching in our waters; oft-times by the mere showing of our presence, so that it was not called for to go a-board. Other-times, Captain Angel (who was after Captain Tindall) would put a Frenchie's boat under arrest in the Name of the King.

"Tor Bay was a most pleasaunt place, and a safe haven, where Captain Angel would go ashore; and I was part of the landing party which went into Briseham and fraterniz'd with the fishers there; and our duty was to find if the fishers were troubled with Frenchies, which they said they were not. But Captain Angel said they might think again if they had not some cause that we should remain in that place for their protection. They 'took his drift' as we were wont to say, and said that they had been hasty, and there was cause to think they might be troubled with Frenchies, so we should stay until we were certain that their waters and creeks were clear.

"We made right merry there, in the inns and taverns of the quayside, and were much favor'd by the Devon Dumplings, which is what the strumpets were call'd thereabouts, and went up upon Borough Head, where we lay in the grass, and I bethought me in paradise, it being so warm and lush and salty, and the sea-gulls crying, and the women so buxom. And, afterward, we crossed the bay on the coast-guard's jolly-boat, the Red-Cliffes of Pampton to larboard, and put ashore at Torre, where there are not so many fishers, but they have storehouses there for salting and for smoking, and the cliffes and the River Flete there brought something of my Jamaican home back to me.

"Through the crossing and the evening at Torre, the Coast-guard made much of staring at me, which I am not un-used to. At last, all un-look'd for, he approach'd me, saying: 'You, Blacky,

Ho there." I replying, he says: 'Name Johnson, Doctor, anything to you?'

"I was sharply taken aback by this, but could not deny my friend and master. "We've had a signal in your regard, 'tis my belief. Can't mind the drift on it, for that it's been a long time since, but I'll wager you'm the subject of it. How be you call'd, boy?'

"'Land-man Barber', I told him swiftley, fearing some ill-tidings from Gough Square.

"'Barber. That's it,' says he. 'Afore ye sail on the morrow, I'll have the paper row'd out to ye,' turning to Captain Angel, 'for as I recall, 'tis come from the highest quarter.'

"Thus did my nautical life find its conclusion. On the following day, still lying off Tor Bay, Captain Angel summoned me to his cabin, whereat he shew'd me a paper from the Admiralty, advising that I must be discharged from the service, Mister Smollett having interceded on the behalf of Doctor Johnson, pleading my youth and a complaint of the throat, which was nothing more than that which formed part of my distemper two years before.

"I wanted none of this; though, when I thought of him, I miss'd the Doctor greatly; but my face was lost among the company and I knew my life there was done.

"Many say that a glimpse of paradise presages the end of life, and was surely so for me in Tor Bay. Forty days follow'd, that were like to waiting for death; for I was no longer enroll'd, and was not one with my companions more, but must stay aboard the Stag for the absolute discharge, which would be at Sheerness.

"I had fallen, once more, into such a low humour that all reason was gone from me. I merely awaited the time when the thing would be done with, thinking to return to Gough Square in defeat, so was surpriz'd, at Sheerness, when instructed to go before the Purser – not having recall'd that there was discharge pay owing above the pittaunce, and I left the captainerye in a much cheerier way.

"I can now confess that, knowing my old master waited to

welcome me back, I made no hurry; taking such time, and such pleasures as my discharge would afford me along the way; until, coming to the house in Gough Square, I found him gone and a new household install'd.

"Now I was in great shame for having taken him for granted, and for having squandered my pay; for which I though his disappearance retribution; so I swore that, if I ever found him more, I should never again desert his friendship, nor quit his service."

CHAPTER FOUR

IN WHICH MASTER BARBER AND YOUR REPORTER EMBARK
UPON A TOUR OF LICHFIELD AND DISCOURSE UPON DIVERS
SUBJECTS, SUCH AS FRIENDSHIP AND JOHNSON'S VIEWS ON
RACE. IN WHICH ALSO IS AN ACCOUNT OF A VISIT TO
DEVONSHIRE AND SOME ANTICKS OF THE DOCTOR'S, AT SEA
AND ASHORE

Our meal having been concluded with a fine cherry-pye, I, feeling the want of air, and interested to see some of those parts of the towne frequented by Doctor Johnson, asked my guest if he would consent to go abroad; in which he acquiesced most readily, so that, when we had attended to our comfort, we left by the street-door and turned to the right, as it were in the direction of London.

After the Market-Street, opposite to which is the way to the Roman Road for Wall, Bird-street runs into St. John's-street, wherein Master Barber identified, upon the right hand, the old Friary, which had housed a body of grey Friars, who had been a force in the towne in the olden tymes, but which was lately the home of Mrs. Cobb and Miss Adey, who were friends of Miss Lucy Porter and of the Doctor, Miss Porter being the daughter of the Doctor's wyfe.

A little way further, we came upon the Hospital of St. John. Here did the Johnson family worship for a time, though not accompanyed by the Young Samuel, when the old spyre of St. Mary's fell down; their pews having been removed hither. The building is at the parting of the ways; that to Birmingham taking the right fork in open mead, the London Road to the left, flanked by the coppices and woodlands of Burrow Hill.

My companion led me across the causeway and out into the country-side, where we climbed a bank, near the crown of which were rankes of cherry-trees, and another church came into view, for which we made. Crossing some stiles, he informed me that these were Levett's Fields, wherein his master had taken great sport in leaping those same stiles, when beyond his sixtieth year

"The fine new towne-house you observe below us, 'twixt the

bakeryes and Tamworth Street, was constructed by Miss Porter. She call'd it Red-Court, tho' I'm told by the common people here that it should be 'Bread-Court'", said he, pointing to a worthy residence in the fashionable taste, the garden being the most pleasing feature thereof, though much obscur'd by an high wall.

Coming out, at last, into the Green-Hill next Rotten Row, which is the way to Tamworth, we took the road for Burton, the fame of whose ale is know'n throughout the land. On a knoll to the right of this road is the church we had espyed across the fields - St Michael's - in whose yard are berryed the mother, father and brother of Johnson.

From this point could be seen, arrayd beneath us, the city and towne; so that we could see all the beauty of it, and could marvell thereon, to see at once all the places of Young Samuel's growing up, and to see how fair was his fortune to be borne in such a place.

On the downes before us, which my companion says are call'd Paradise!, and down about the pools, people of all kinds disported themselves, lounging, reading, running, taking sustenaunce and playing at games with stick and ball, many among them trades-people and their familyes, taking of their ease upon the Lord's Day.

Espying a flowrye tussock, which had seem'd to be lay'd there for the purpose, we took our part with the others in that idyllick scene, and sprawled likewise upon the warm verdaunce.

"Such rustick magnificence is highly priz'd by a London-Man such as I am," I observed. "Contemplation of the beautyes of Nature being such a diversion and a healing thing, with sunlight and good-aires to breathe and the workes of our Maker in trew evidaunce, I must *love* this favour'd land, and recall the reasons why we busy ourselves in the filthy burrowes of the Capital for its profit and protection."

"I must own to sharing your rural predilection, Master Reporter; for I find that, as well as repose, such commerce with the stuff of nature aids also the development of true wisdom, and comprehension of the forces to which we are subject, and which we might come to tame."

"A lofty thought, sir, but I'm not agin it."

"Few knew more of the lofty than my late master; but rustick idyll was naught to him. He'd as lief taken this fine view of his old home as not, the mean and airless courts of 'the needy villain's gen'ral home' being much more to his liking. Indeed, it oft seem'd to me that he would become morose and frantick if deny'd his just portion of squalour. The filth and the dregs of the stinking dens and rookeryes, he marshall'd for his ideas and his poetry. The only *natural* thing for which he had any affection was people, and these in all shapes and forms; though young women being his particular preference." This was the second occasion upon which he had produc'd a strange leer in his master's connexion.

We being well-found on our soft and springye bank, I took the moment to direct him back to his storye:

"So the menage in Gough Square was disbanded, you say."

"That it was, and much else had changed during my Sea-Life, including that he had been twice to Oxford, since leaving that house, and had also caus'd the petition to go forward for my dis-charge a full one and one-half years before I had receiv'd notice of it.

"He was otherwise alone, having been much reduc'd of circumstaunce, and having no need of a house the size of Gough Square, so had moved first to lodgings in Staple's Inn, follow'd by something of the same in Gray's Inn; but, on my enquiring his whereabouts of Mister Strahan, the printer, I was told to look for him upon the first floor of the house at number one Inner Temple Lane, next the corner shoppe, on the river-side of Fleet Street.

"Which is where I found him; and, having once done so, never lost him more until it would be forever, or until I am permitted to join him."

'Permitted' seem'd an odd word here, but I chose not to take it up with him for the moment.

"We embrac'd, I think, for the first time, truly as friends, for we both wish'd to be where we were, and that the other be with us there. He ask'd to hear all about my life at sea, which I told him, and thank'd him for his love and friendship in seeking my dis-charge and bringing me to the attention of such as Mister Wilkes, who was near the highest in the land, and I swore to him that I would never more desert him, to which he replied the same to me; which touch'd us both, so that we fell a-blubbing out of control. Then he bade me kneel by him, and composed a prayer of thanks-giving and of supplication that we might continue thus.

"What follow'd was to be the most joyous period of my life with him, being two years in which we should be un-troubled by Williams and the rest, and I should receive of much attention from him."

"I'm surpriz'd to hear you describe your-selves as 'friends', for you were surely 'master' and 'servant', or, perhaps, 'master' and 'companion'. It is difficult to think that such a relationship can permit this usage."

I did not wish, having had my own opinions throw'n in disarray by the singular nature of Master Barber, to refer to assertions that Johnson regarded the negro races as inferiors, so could not have accepted this idea, but I must put forth some challenge for his answer.

"There was nothing in the character or opinion of the Doctor that should preclude it, sir. Though each should know his station, and discharge the duties thereof, that station, whether it concern the compiling of a dictionary, or the preparation of a supper, is as much part of the net-work of life. Those who undertake useful activity are to be respected as fellow-humans, or as nothing. Mister Boswell, for all that I love him, and that he has been a friend to me in life, has written that my late master believed in the inferiority of some races.

"In this, as in some other things, he was simply mis-taken. My master's view was shar'd with his much older friend, the poet, Mister Richard Savage, who was a free-thinker, and wrote the lines:

'Why must I Afric's sable Children see
'Vended for Slaves, though form'd by Nature free,
'The nameless Tortures cruel Minds invent,
'Those to subject, whom Nature equal meant?'

"If only what is reported of Doctor Johnson's own speech be read, a fair indication of his real opinions may be had, but Mister Boswell finds him oblig'd to super-impose his own views upon the issue, which is not the work of a biographer, but part of his own desire for fame and literary im-mortality, as any who know him will readily cognite.

"Doctor Johnson was my friend, I say again; and I his — he, thereafter all-ways addressing me as 'Frank' and, in our private doings, I alone call'd him 'Doctor Sam', and I would tolerate what-ever other reverses might come, knowing that fact alone - that Doctor Samuel Johnson was Francis Barber's friend."

"I must stand corrected by you, sir, and can readily see how it could be so. I hope you will allow my ignorance, and favour me with the continuation of your history." I had not commenced upon that day with the thought of having my ideas of the world tried, let alone that they should be so put about that I could not yet fix my opinions on what I had heard; and I knew that I should yet hear more from this singular personage that would test my wits.

However, I was by no means inclined to pro-crastination, as you may be sure, since I must be returned to London by the evening of the twenty-second, which was the morrow. So I must hear all he had to say, though I might meditate upon it at leisure thereafter.

"The new King (George III) was crown'd while I was at sea, and he was desireous of fostering more of the artistick and litterary than had been to his predecessor's taste, to which end he granted the Royal Society of Arts in Covent Garden, Mister Reynolds being put in charge thereof.

"My master had delivered his *Rasselas*, and was occupied upon divers dedications and reviews, but could not claim 'pecuniary inexigency', as I once heard him describe it.

Unbeknownst to him, some of his friends had advanced a proposal that he might be given support, in the form of a reward or pension in recognition of his merit and achievements.

"It is well that they did not inform him of the proposal in advance of its realisation, as he had succumbed to one of his caprices when defining of the word in his Dictionary. A *'pension'*, so he said, was 'an allowance made to any one without an equivalent', by which he meant a payment for which nothing was given in return, a process he found abhorrent in the extreme, which was at the core of his hatred of the stock-jobbers, who prov'd his point in the *South Seas* affair.

"But he could not credit that the King or the Parliament would pay money from the exchequer for nothing, so added the more shocking assertion that 'in England it is generally understood to mean pay given to a state hireling for treason to his country', no doubt with a particular instance in mind, though he never communicated the details in my hearing.

"Though he had not been instrumental, nor even privvy, to the securing of it, still he had a difficulty about its acceptaunce, for that it would seem that his lexicography must apply to all but him-self. Accordingly, he determined to ask for *advice*, though he was never much for listening to that commodity, and was really seeking *encouragement*, the money being greatly needed, and he having not the merest thought of turning it down!

"He went for this 'advice' to Mister Reynolds, a firm and honest friend, not without experience of Royal patronage, hence well-fitted to supply a true *picture* of the responsibilities of such a benefice. As in his *portraits*, he put the subject in its *best light*, and my master was soon writing in gracious acceptaunce.

"The pension was fix'd at three hundred pounds per annum — a not in-considerable amount for a lesson I had already learn'd for twelve. But he was in great joy and gratitude, and I with him, for he saw that financial pressures were eas'd and, since he ever claim'd that none but a blockhead would bother to write but for money, he lay'd down his pen at once.

"He made much of the rise of Mister — or Sir Joshua, as he now was — Reynolds, saying such things as 'he now charges twenty guineas a head,' or 'he continues to add thousands to thousands,' so it was in this spirit that he announc'd that we should be going with him to Devon, 'to enable Sir Joshua's teller to catch up on the accounting, while he is temporarily removed from further escalation of the reckoning.'.

"For my part, I could envisage nothing better than returning to Devon in the company of my master, and he was in high anticipation, following Sir Joshua's and my own descriptions of the place."

"Doctor Johnson had never been to Devon." This was an observation of the obvious on my part, but was more a spoken thought than a point for discussion.

"At that point in his life, sir, though he had much to say upon the subject, he had never seen the sea! The entirety of his material universe was from Lichfield to London, by way of Birmingham and Oxford. Beyond this was the universe of his intellect, which was boundless; though parts of it vye-ing with the material for immutability."

"You are sharp with your late master's foibles, sir," I rallied.

"I had the best teacher; and 'tis ever the sharpness of affection. Only the truly great can be precisely described, without recourse to hollowe flatterye or varnish. My Johnson suffer'd no fools, and brought me up in his method, which hath not all-ways brought me patron-age, but has ever exempted me from patron-ising'"

"Bravo, sir. Prittily said." I wav'd him on.

"I don't know if you can imagine with what emotions, with what sense of wonder, a person of low birth, accustomed to a squalid existence, either at sea or in London, comes upon the Stately houses of England. I was so much in awe of those we visited on this 'jaunt', of which there were several, that I was as in a dream, and awaking, could recall little of detail about them.

"We were at Hawldon, Coat-Hill, Saltram and others, which were so large your master might never find you, and which afforded numerous opportunities for the improuvement of my knowledge, particularly with respect to dairy-maids.

"We went also to Plymouth, which was marvellous for its ships and docks and all things to do with the Navy. I was in my own element in the Dock-yard, and amus'd the Doctor and Sir Joshua with my enthousiastick explanations of all that was there to be seen.

"Then a messenger came, bearing the compliments of the Dock-yard Commissioner, requesting the pleasure of Doctor Johnson and Sir Joshua Reynolds's companye, and offering to convey them in his yaghte to visit the light-tower lately built by Smeaton upon the Eddy-stone; to which they readily and gratefully consented, though I was fearful, sensing a change in the wind and aire, which I was sure betray'd a gathering storm."

"A-ha,' Know you aught of meteorology, sir?"

"Meteor-ology? The examination of shooting-stars; a study speedily concluded." This was blatant parody.

"No, sir. Rather: the observation and prediction of climatic processes, the word deriving from the Greek, *meta* — about, after or concerning; and, *aeiro* — air, or, more literally, raise; with *logos* — (suggestive of study and discourse) the word, hence —*ology*, (qv)."

"You speak sooth, master Reporter, though mine was more Johnsonian. My reply to your inquiry is to say that a sea-going man who knows naught of the observation and prediction of climatic processes is in a fair way of finding him-self speedily concluded! Though he may have none of books and learning, the matelot can read the wind, or he could never rig a sail; and his lessons are his scorch'd skin, his contusions, his weals and his blisters, which he has by heart and want for no re-vysing. If you would know aught of meteor-ology, sir, cast away books and consult a sea-farer, I say."

I began to find this a little over-done, so, lest I come to regret my pleasaunt inquiry, I cried finish: "How took bold Johnson to his first encounter with that other element, I'd like to know?"

"Right *boldly*, sir. Indeed, most surprizingly so. 'Twas second-nature to *me*, and Sir Joshua, being a Devon man, was a sea-dog born; but, whereas all of us others on board were respectful and trepidacious of our being at the mercy of so great a power, the Doctor took the celestial side.

"Our crossing of what is call'd the Sound commenced in a calm enough way, being in the lee of Mount-Edge-Come, but the stirrings I had felt a-shore soon grew into a full-blow'n tempest, and, though we came within an half-cable of the Eddy-Stone, the captain must cry 'Avast,' or see us dasht to pieces.

"Not in the slightest degree discomfited by this, the Doctor strode about the heaving deck, a-waving of his arms, and crying the cause of turbulence, as the spray soak'd him and the waves crash'd about him. 'Unleash thy worst!' 'Show us thy extremity!' 'Boil, ye depths!' 'Try us with all thy might and main!' - these and other such exhortations did he offer, revelling in the tumult."

"He was un-doubtedly a most singular personage," I had to own. Boswell refers to some similar anticks in Scotch waters, in the course of their travells in those regions. I, myself, have oft witness'd strange behaviour by people out of their element, but never such as is attributed to Johnson. "What made the companye of such a spectacle?" I wonder'd.

"For all that they be oaken-hearted, seamen were ever superstitious, so did not find the Doctor's challenges much to their liking, I think, for we were not ask'd if we would stay and regard Mister Smeaton's light-tower from there. Orders were giv'n and we made for the shore. It's my belief that they mark'd the Doctor as a *jonah*."

"Is it not to be wonder'd at that, in our age of reason, such superstitions persist in being held, when Men of Science have taken such pains to dis-credit them? Should not the un-Scientifick be excluded from His Majesty's Service?" This I thought to be un-contentious rhetorick, having not yet fully learn'd that Master Barber's education under Doctor Johnson did not permit of such a thing.

"Never, sir. Truth is not a dogmatic assertion, but something waiting to be found out. Reason is the means of that finding-out, and is as good as it is free to function. The reason of our age suffers already from being bound to particular disciplines.

"The placing of those things which do not fit our fashionable models beyond the law is not reasonable, especially when those same things existed previous to our modern sciences and persist in the face of them, for they are not answer'd by being declar'd illegitimate.

"If reason be limited by earthly authority, it is surely reason no more. As *Hamlet* said: 'There are more things in heaven and earth, Horatio, than are dreamt of in your philosophy.'. Those that would wish to impose *stasis* upon th'unruly and *kinetic* by no other means than authour-ized declaration, would do better to repeat the words of the Bard.

"The Earl of Orrery was a frequent visiter to Gough Square in the old days. If you have seen the devyse which bears his name, you will readily see that the mariner's superstition, which allows of un-earthly influences, albeit im-perfectly, or un-Scientifickally identifyed, is more comprehensive than the dogma of the Newtonian, which permits of nothing not observ'd, decided upon and elabourated by other Newtonians.

"If authorities upon the world of the sea exist, they are those who live by and on it. Others may measure it, observe it and test its propertyes; but their maps, their charts, their records and their formulae, even if all put together, still are not the sea, but merely observations upon it."

"Was Mister Smeaton's light-tower worth the *crossing* of it, *I'd* like to know."

"Faith, sir, that it was, being truly a marvell of the modern world. How came those gigantick, and perfectly cut stones to that desolate rock, how put ashore, and how constructed in such smooth fashion, I cannot en-visage. The light with which it sweeps the sea must be provided with oil in like manner. In the cruel seas of mid-winter, the light-men must be the loneliest men alive."

"And what thought your master and his friend?"

"The Doctor referr'd to it not at all, being engag'd upon his gyrations from the time it hove into view until it was lost from us.

"Sir Joshua was much excited by the prospect, bidding all who would listen to him observe the quality of light upon the sky, the singularity of the reflections upon the cylindrick walls of the tower, and the corruscations proceeding from the motion of the waves, the while holding of his thumb before him, regarding and pro-portioning the scene therewith, as it were a victim in his studio.

"I'm sure he believ'd that he would make a painting of it when he was re-united with his brushes; but I'd be equally prepar'd to wager that he never did, he being not much for things that won't sit, still as the grave before him, for hours together.

"No, not a painter of motion, Sir Joshua. Preferr'd subjects: titled and paralytick!

"A new towne had grown up around the Dock-yard to accommodate the dockers and other persons there employ'd, with the result that a spirit of competition and controversy had arisen between this place and the established towne and city of Plymouth, two miles distant.

"The new towne wanted a supplye of water, a commodity of which Plymouth had more than enough, the surplus running away into the sea. I believe it had been brought thither by some feat of engineering, which in that land of hills and coombes would be requir'd, but that the supply was warranted to be of consistent amount and quality.

"The following day, the storm having blow'n over, we were upon the Barbican when we came up with a party of politickers who were giving forth how the new towne was trying to usurp the place of Plymouth, and pouring every sort of scorn upon the dockers there and all their works.

"A look, with which I was more than familiar, came into the Doctor's good eye, and I was sure that he meant to enter into the contro-versy, it being his practice ever to take the contrary position in all discussion. A smile from Sir Joshua told me that he was in on the game.

"But our Johnson was in an especially fine humour, and minded to be more contrary still; doing the opposite to that which we anticipated, and falling in with the politickers.

"'I am a *Plymouth* man' he averr'd, 'and I am against the dockers. Let the rogues die of thirst, before they have any of *our* good *Plymouth* water.' He was having splendid sport, and gathered a good crowd about him, repeating his harangues ever louder. Finally, in a confiding way, he lean'd toward those at the front of the on-lookers and said: 'I *hate* a docker,' occasioning much mirth, which continued behind us as we mov'd on.

"He oftentimes used the word, 'hate', but all-ways in a most singular fashion, for I believe that he never truly hated any one, considering such an emotion ridiculeous and un-reasonable. When-ever he profess'd to hate some one or some thing, as I was to learn, it was to draw forth an examination of a commonly held prejudice.

"For me, this was an early key to the subtilty of his character, for he call'd Doctor Bathurst 'a good *hater*', which I, at first, found most perplexing; but later understood the jest, at which I commenc'd upon the long road to understanding Doctor Johnson.

"He did another singular thing while we were at Plymouth. He and Sir Joshua were the house-guests of the chirurgeon, Doctor Mudge, a worthy good man of exquisite manners, and among the company was a woman, who I think was one of the Misses Parker. She, being a great admirer of Doctor Johnson, was full of in-form'd questions for him upon his work.

"He was ever particularly pleas'd with female attention, more especially as on this occasion, when it took the form of un-alloy'd admiration, so was responding to each of her points in a serious and comprehensive fashion.

"She then turn'd to the subject of the Dictionary, inquiring as to why he had defin'd *'pastern'* (being that part of a horse's foot between the hoof and the fettlock) as 'the *knee* of an horse'.

"Un-hesitatingly, and with the same gravity that had attended his earlier responses, he replied: 'Ignorance, madam; pure ignorance'.

"He afterward told me that he had greatly enjoy'd his 'Devon jaunt' it having furnish'd the stuff of many new ideas."

CHAPTER FIVE

IN WHICH THE BIOGRAPHER, BOSWELL, ENTERS THE
NARRATIVE; IS PARODIED BY MASTER BARBER AND CALLED
'IDLE' BY THE DOCTOR; AND WE BEGIN TO APPREHEND
SOMETHING OF OUR SUBJECT'S CONDITION

"We return'd to Inner Temple Lane to find Doctor Levet married and ill-tidings of Doctor Bathurst."

"Your life at that time would appear to have been much populated by Doctors,"I observed, "Levet, Bathurst, Mudge, Johnson...."

"Quite so, sir, and there's not much alteration now with respect to that; but *our* Doctor, whom Johnson and I valued above all others, was then lost to us.

"Doctor Bathurst (Doctor *Richard*, as he shall ever be to me) had tried without success to establish a practice in London of sufficient extent to support him and his houses there and in the Cathedral Close at Lincoln, where I had been in his late father's service. He had decided, therefore, to go for an army physician, and had perish'd at the Havannah, which a-griev'd us very much."

"What work was Johnson engaged upon at that time?"

"He was still about his reviews and dedications, the only one of which I recall being for the artists' exhibition. He had not yet commenced upon his *Shakespeare*, as I remember. It was around that time that he met Mister Boswell for the first time at Mister Davies, the bookseller's house, at Russell Street, Covent Garden.

"From the start, it was evident that Mister Boswell much admir'd the Doctor, and wish'd to cultivate his friendship, which was not uncommon among writers of all kinds, but my Master (contrarily, as ever was, with his professed opinions of the Scotch) was quite taken with him in turn, and encourag'd his attention They met upon several occasions at the *Mitre*, and stay'd quite late.

"A few weeks after their first meeting, Mister Boswell invited the Doctor to dine with him in his lodgings in Downing

Street, but arriv'd that morning, in an agitated condition, at Inner Temple Lane, which was the first time I had set eyes upon him myself.

"Until he told me who he was, I could not have guess'd it, for he was very young, puppy-ish, you might say and was in such an excitement that I took him not seriously. 'Ah, Frank,' he said, 'I must see your master at once!'

"Later, I would come to like and admire him very well, and to *enjoy* the sudden-ness of his address, for he was never much giv'n to social flummery; but, upon this occasion, I took him to be an uncouth lunatick. 'I believe you to be mis-taken in that regard, sir,' I truth-fully advised him, and closed the street-door; at which he took up such a terrible rapping with his metall'd stick that I must open to him again. 'Frank, I'm sure your master will see me.'.

"His familiar use of my name was not something I could easily accept, each instance affecting, for the worse, my disposition toward him. 'If I am to put your conviction to the test, I shall be forced to identify its possessor; in which, sir, you have the advantage of me.'.

"On hearing this, he bow'd low, doffing his odd little bonnet: 'James Boswell, Esquire, at your service,' says he; whereon I inform'd him that what-ever description he had had of *me* was better than any I had of *him*, and went to consult the Doctor, who did, indeed, agree to see him at once.

"It turn'd out that there had been some altercation with his land-lord, which necessitated his speedy removal; though he was more concern'd about his inability to honour his supper invitation, than he was about his own domiciliary inadequacy.

"Now fairly may it be said of the dear Doctor that, when he was up, he was up, and when he was down, he was down! He had been in a terrible affliction when first I came to Gough Square, and remain'd so for a long time after the death of Mrs. J., but had afterward recover'd his humours to a mark'd degree. He had been similarly terrourized for some time previous to my return from the sea, coming to himself so much thereafter, most part-icularly in the period of the Devon Jaunt, that hardly a thing could be seen to try him; he remaining in the best mood, regardless of all about him.

"So it was that, refusing to display either shock or sympathye to poor Mister Boswell in his extremity, he made it plain that he consider'd the entire business a subject for mirth, sorely trying the Scotchman's temper by telling him to consider how insignificant it would be a twelvemonth thence.

"At last, however, he was able to calm him, agreeing to be his guest at the *Mitre*, with Mister Davies, Mister Goldsmith and others."

"The great biographer did not much impress you on that occasion, then, that you gave him such a reception."

"It was my duty to turn away interlopers and unwelcome callers. When my master was at his writing he could be more than a little displeas'd with disturbance; which, if I had not prevented, I might have been the cause of.

"For aught I knew, Boswell was a young rake, come to make sport with my master, or with me. It should not have been the first such occurrence, were it so."

"I have the image of him as a dour and humour-less individual, all awe and attention toward your master (and any other man of merit), but rather stolid and plodding in his way. I had not thought of his ever having been young, so am interested by your first impressions of him." I was keen to form a picture of the man I now knew to be ailing and withdrawn from society, by the report of someone who had known him 'in the flesh', as the saying is.

"You must have come to know him very well," said I. "What was he like?"

Not without some difficulty, my companion came to his feet, and commenc'd to walk about before me in a manner aberrated and prissy, a-smoothing of his coat. "D'ye not think ma new coat the very THING, mon?" he demanded in the coarsest Scotch accents, his dark countenaunce and shabby cloathes according his personation even greater absurdity. "D'ye not think it flatters my manly form? D'ye not think I cut something of a figure? All the bloods and rakes must stand aside this night, for

Beau Boswell will have his choice of the ladyes. I've a parcel of Mrs. Phillips's cundums in ma pocket - so, when ma new coat and ma manly bearing warms 'em, and my size inflame's 'em, 'twill be aye pleasure and nae consequences.'"

He deliver'd this last with a wink and a grotesque flourish. Then, holding one hand aloft, he plac'd of the other upon his hip and began to cavort about on tip-toe, the while bursting forth a second time in song, if so it may be call'd:

Yeer eyes are like the burns i' Spring;
Yeer voice the Summer breeze;
And, when I see yeer wee mooth smile,
I fa' upon ma knees.

Wul ye gi' me o' yeer fern-red hair
T' pu' i'side ma lockit?
F' there is nae lass which can surpass
Sweet Meg o' Drumnadrochit."

Finishing, he bow'd low and fell back upon the grass. "That, sir, was James Boswell to the life; *that* your serious and stolid biographer. He lov'd Johnson, he lov'd women, and he lov'd himself, which may have been the order of precedence; for, if the first were not available, he would be about the second; if neither the first, nor the second, he was ever well-satisfied with the third.

"But he had a childlike spirit, with a sense of wonder and a desire for pleasure which never could be quenched, and he was ever honest, which qualities I much lik'd him for. I think 'twas also these attributes which interested the Doctor, for he was more tolerant with him than with any other man, allowing him access to his very soul, which the deluded Knight had not come within an hundred miles of."

This was a reference to Johnson's other biographer, Sir John Hawkins, who, as Master Barber's narrative was to reveal, was wanting in a number of relations.

"Also, though he could be dour and melancholick, as you

suggest, he was the more often a truly merry fellowe, much giv'n to singing and dauncing in a manner entirely spontaneous. He gave out that he was a 'most excellent man', which, in his innocent and light-hearted way, few took amiss, and most ended by believing. Only those over-burden'd with their own import persisted in thinking him an ideot, though I'll own 'twas an easy first impression!

"He did well by my Master; and, after *he* was gone, did well by me. I will hear nothing but good of him, and gave that personation in a spirit of love, knowing that he would have taken no offence from it.

"Indeed, had he seen it, I should surely have made a life's work of it, for he was an untiring enthousiast for anything of which he was at the centre.

'Mister Boswell was also the only man I ever knew who was not en-slav'd by money. His income came to him as some form of allowance from his father, who was a Scotch Laird, but he was able to accept owner-ship easily, and to value it in the terms of his own needs and requirements. By a system that was uniquely his own, he would save money by quibbling over accomm-odations or victuals, while un-questioningly paying the asking price to tailors and harlots.

"His allowance was not without conditions, but he turn'd these to his own use, claiming an intention to join the Guards as his reason for being in London, so that His Laird-ship would, all un-witting, support his drinking and whoring. Then 'twas got wind of, so, some two or three months after he and my Master met, he must take the expedient of going to the Low Countryes to study the law, which his father wish'd for him, being in that way him-self.

"The Doctor never lik'd to be parted from company, especially if 'twere as agreeable as he found Mister Boswell; but I never, before or since, knew him to go to such trouble as he did at that time to procure the last possible *drop* of companion-ship from any one.

"It was his invariable practise to accompany visiters to the stair, usually going with them to the street-door. More often than not, he would escort them to their carriage, or, if afoot, out into the main thoroughfare; the more when we liv'd in the courts.

"When it came time for Mister B.'s departure, he accompanyed him all the way to Har'ich in the stage-coach, a round-trip of nigh-on two hundred miles, so that he must pass the night at Coalchester; and they had a tender parting, vowing to spend more time in company at the conclusion of his (Boswell's) legal apprehensions.

"Mister Boswell later gave an account of the journey to Har'ich, which you may have read. The Doctor was not much for anecdote, so I often learnt more about his sayings and doings from others, being frequently remouv'd from their actual playing out.

"According to Mister Boswell, one of their fellow-passengers was an old fat-woman. When they stopt at an inn for dinner, this woman spoke at some length how she had taken great pains to educate her children, having never suffer'd them to be idle. The Doctor, upon finishing his meal, (for he never spoke while eating), said: 'I wish, Madam, you would educate me too; for I have been an idle fellow all my life.'

"'I am sure you have not been idle,' the woman reply'd.

"'Nay, Madam, it is very true; and that gentleman *there*, (pointing at Mister B.), has been idle. He was idle at Edinburgh. His father sent him to Glasgow, where he continued to be idle. He then came to London, where he has been very idle; and now he is going to Utrecht, where he will be as idle as ever.'

"At the time, Mister Boswell thought this to be un-supportable ridicule, believing of him-self materially reduc'd by the Doctor's triflings; but he was later able to tell it against him-self, which show'd that he had learnt one of the lessons my Master lik'd most to teach (albeit he never perfectly learnt it him-self)"

"I may be a jot slow, but I cannot see the lesson in't at once."

"Why, it is that the significance of a thing lies not within the thing, but is attach'd to it in the observation. The actuality that was James Boswell, the conception he had of him-self, was, in no degree, alter'd by the Doctor's skit upon him. This, at least, was what the Doctor contended.

"The woman would retain an image of Boswell as 'an idle fellowe', perhaps; but, if the Doctor had said *naught*, she might have recall'd him as 'plump', 'ill-favour'd' or 'nasally predominant'. What of it?"

"Ah. I take the point."

"But, of course, there is another way of looking at it. In a sense, Mister Boswell *was* chang'd by the suggestion that he was un-remittingly idle, in that he took offense against it and believ'd him-self wounded. Though the Doctor past it off by telling him that the woman would think of him no more thereafter, I don't believe that this was reassuraunce to a man in search of posteritye, such as Boswell was. Indeed, if he wanted to be no more thought of in that character, why did he ensure its writing-down and eternal repetition?

"The real lesson Boswell learnt was that the man who laughs *with* the world will not be laugh'd at *by* it."

"You say that Johnson could not learn his own lesson."

"Nor could he, sir. Much has been said of the Doctor's melancolick propensityes. He was much a-fear'd of letting madness in, believing it to be ever attendant upon him; so, whilst he was happy to display the folly of others, and to make fun of their characters, he could not easily accept any criticism or ragging himself.

"Though it ever went contrary to his reason, and his advanc'd views, he could but rarely permit others to pierce his certainty. He could take opposing or novel views from a book, for he was in control of the book, and the reading of it; but an opposing view advanc'd without he was pre-par'd for it, in publick, often met with compleat annihilation.

"While he retain'd control, all was well. At the suggestion he might be losing it, he would fight his corner better than Mendoza.

"Fear ever causes us to with-draw our perception; and his fear blinded him to that very control with which he was obsess'd, so that an inexorable and subtile change supervened, that he had not the slightest inkling of.

"Whereas he continued to see himself as Master, with Mister Boswell as pupil and willing slave; the latter had the advantage that he put the Doctor's teachings into practice, which, habitually, the Doctor did not.

"By degrees, therefore, the precedence was alter'd; the perspicaceous pupil learning to be master; and the trusting master meta-morphosing into a subject of biography, where once he had been his own man.

"Boswell used him as well as any man might; but *that* he used him, there can be no doubt, not limiting himself to that personal selection of traits and doings which must constitute all biography, (be they selected by motive, ignorance, or memory), but contriving, as far as possible, the scenes and topicks of it in advance.

"As he owns in his 'Dedication to Sir Joshua', he has been at pains to preclude a recurrence of the mis-takes of *his* character which had been caus'd by the publick taking his account of the Doctor's joshings in his Tour of the Hebrides too literally, by choosing not to give as compleat an account in his 'Life'.

"If he has form'd *himself* into that which he believes will attract publick approbation, what will he not do, when it is his to dictate, with the life of his *hero?*

"Near the end the Doctor instructed me to destroy his own accounts of parts of his life, which I did not do; for, despite all of Mister Boswell's efforts for candour, in those alone was he fully himself, rather than an inevitably imperfect copy.

"There, and in his other written work, does he truly survive; though Boswell, Mrs. Piozzi, yea, and even the Knight preserve memories of him.

"Those of great repute are ever re-moulded for the ends of chroniclers and historians. Samuel Johnson can give a good account of *himself.*

"Those whose tenuous connexion to repute may bring them contagious transmutation are not, as a rule, possessed of such protection.

CHAPTER SIX

IN WHICH REPORTER AND SUBJECT ARE SOMEWHAT AFFECTED BY THE LOCAL CYDER AND FRANCIS TELLS HOW HE WAS TOUCHED BY LOVE IN LINCOLNSHIRE

The excellent dinner we had taken at the Swan had, for some time, been growing heavy upon me, induceing some measure of somnolence.

I must have been o'erwhelm'd by it at last, for, when I came next to myself, I could not immediately descry Master Barber.

I thought to go in search of him, but, sure that he would return in due course, and thinking that way to miss him, I sat up and gaz'd across the meadow, which was now reddening in the afternoon sunlight.

At length, I espied the figure of my companion, coming from a track to the north-east; in his hand, a flagon of cyder, which, as he came nigh, he held aloft: "Halloo, master Reporter. I bring refreshment. I talk'd too much and sent you to sleep, so I make amends with the best cyder to be had hereabouts, warranted to moisten your tongue, and fortifye your ears !"

I took a swig, right gratefully, and assured him, at once, that 'twas but the heavy dinner and want of refreshment that had brought about my lapse; that I was now restor'd and avid to hear more of his account, as soon as he should feel ready to continue.

"Mister Boswell remain'd abroad for a considerable time - two years and more - during which time he completed his studyes at Utrecht and rambled around Europe, visiting Italy, Sardinia, Corsica and France, in which last he met with Monsure Voltair.

"He and the Doctor wrote letters to each other the while, and they shar'd some evenings at the Mitre upon his return. But he did not stay long, for he must return to Scotchland to practice the laws that he had learn't upon his travels, and for which his Laird-ship had pay'd.

"So, all-in-all, he was five years away."

"Did Johnson keep to London in his absence?"

"No, sir. We were soon off to Lincolnshire, though not to the city of Lincoln, where I had previously liv'd but to the estate of Benet Langton, near Spillsby, which I remember for its treacherous winding roads that threaten'd at every moment to turn the coach over, or throw us in the ditch; the ditches thereabouts being full of water, and capable of drowning a man!

"Mister Langton was young, but an old friend of the Doctor's. He was a very learned man, who, I believe had been taught by someone of the Doctor's acquaintance. I don't now recall the detail. However, Mister Langton had come in search of Doctor Johnson in the early days, when he was still at a loss after the death of Mrs J., and he had also brought Mister Beauclerk, who was a wild person.

"Though they were all so different of age and temper, still they lik'd each other very well, the Doctor being much amus'd by the anticks of Mister Beauclerk, and gratify'd to have, in Mister Langton, a young companion capable of rewarding conversation.

"Mister L. had also an house at Rochester, but his seat was in Lincolnshire, where it had been a goodlye time, to my late Master's delight, he frequently telling how the Langton family went back to King John's day, which was easy to-believe of Old Mister Langton, who seem'd not to have gather'd much since, and took Doctor Johnson for a Roman Catholick!"

"A house such as his must have been well supply'd with servants. Did you find sufficient to occupy you there?"

"Aye, sir. In and out of the house. I was never a man that wanted for amusement, though it might need a bit of a walk to find, and though the snow be upon the ground as it then was.

"Whilst the Doctor and Mister Langton went by coach to Lincoln, I betook myself, with one of Mister Langton's footmen, to Alford market, by which were more inns and ale-houses than I ever saw in such a concentration, and where the local country folk made them right merry.

"The footman was as tall as the Doctor, and a most excellent fellow, well known in Alford, where they were wont to call him

'Long Tom' or it could have been 'Lang Tom', with their rude accents, which play with the name 'Langton', they never ceas'd to find comickal. Arriving together that day, we caus'd something of a sensation, as you might imagine: Long Tom and Dusky Frank, come about some quaffing, with an eye for the local women-kind.

"To say we was successful, in both regards, would not be to overstate it, sir. 'Twas a day to remember, the ale being of the finest, and the local maids vye-ing for our attentions, which led to something of a rumpus with some farm-hands, and our precipitate departure – an incomparable end to an exquisite day!"

"As you say. If 'twere less elevating than your master's, your day o'ertops his for distractions, to be sure. I'm all for un-complicated pleasure such as may be found in rural areas. 'Twere better to be monk-like in London, where an insignificant encounter may leave a mark upon a man out of proportion to its pleasure." Master Barber made me wistful of my youthfull days.

"I'faith, we both bear evidence that, at a pinch, pleasure will win the day, sir." 'Twas true. His black skin bore the signs of the small-pox, though the effect was not so immediate as it is upon the white.

"The revells of that day were not entirely without complication, neither.

"The following morning, the Doctor and Mister Langton went to see Louth, and I stay'd behind at the Hall. I spent the day in telling tales of Jamaica and the pirates thereabouts (which were not of my experience, but mainly from what I had been told by my ship-mates on the Stag), and in teaching the pot-boy how to catch fish in the estate-stream, which was a contributory of the River Steeping.

"When we return'd to the kitchen, they told me I had a caller, which mystify'd me greatly, but they could not keep the smiles from off their faces, so I deem'd that they were playing a jape upon me.

"Prepar'd to take the trick in good part, I went to the parleur, but found there one of the farm girls which had been the subject of the riot the previous day.

"She was a sweet girl, with a natural bloom, and well-made; and she was diff'rent from the others, for, though that she was proud and strong, she was also gentle and soft-spoke, and possess'd of much intelligence. Her eyes, sir, I will not attempt to describe, but that they were deep and pure and honest, and gaz'd at me in a way I had never been (or thought to be) gaz'd upon - I swear it makes me weak to think on them, even now.

"And her voice, sir, what can I say of that? Only that it was the tend'rest voice that ever spoke, or so I thought at that time, and that it was such a voice as set every corporeal thing a-shiver.

"It had been so brave of her to approach that huge house alone, and she had trudged there for no purpose but to see me, which softened my heart, so I could think of nothing but her.

"In my nautical life, I had learn't to take pleasure from women (aye, and to give it), but all casually and with no thought of deeper emotion. 'Twas expedient and lightly done - and none the worse for that - but it gave me no preparation for this occurrence, in which I was a lost man ere I began.

"In short, sir, I had been touch'd by LOVE.

"For all that my body scream'd to possess her, my spirit wanted to enfold and protect her; aye; even from her own folly in pursuing me!

"What she had seen in me - a thoughtless, ill-educated African - that set her in my direction, I never did comprehend. Some talk of a chymystry which influences desire, and it may be true in the matter of carnal lusts.

"But she look'd from beyond her body and I know she saw beyond mine, so that she would have found my appearaunce beautiful if it were not (which, at that time, you may rely upon my assurance that it was)." Here he preen'd himself in a grotesque gesture, which added no conviction to his assuraunce, you may be sure.

"And, strange though I found it (for, in my youthfull ignorance, I believ'd myself a man of the world, fully experience'd in matters of the heart). I regarded her: likewise, being hopelessly smitten and, for the remainder of our time at Langton, being never parted from her but she occupy'd all my thoughts, so that the Doctor bethought me sick.

"If love be a sickness, then I am far gone with it, I told him; which he, at first, thought to be comical; but, when I persisted, became angry, telling me it was nonsense. I was, he told me, not yet fully-form'd; he having plans to this end which would not admit of a dependent (and, which, of course, he would not suffer to be alter'd).

"He told me it was my duty to him (which I had already vow'd to put above all things), and to the girl, to put her off before it went too far, which, for all that I lov'd her, I could see the reason of, she being little vers'd in the ways of the world, so having no idea of what she would be bringing upon herself, by throwing in he lot with the likes of me, a man whose life was still not his; all of which I had told her from the first, with not the slightest effect."

"It must have gone hard on you, but you shew'd maturity and common sense above your years in seeing that the Doctor was right," I put in, for he was dwelling upon the matter, with that far-off look once more in his eyes.

"In that, at least, aye; though not in my treatment of her; for I could not bring myself to tell her. It would have gone so hard with us both, and I was sure she would persuade me to break my vow and remain with her there. If it weren't for the vow, 'twould certainly have been the way of it.

"I thought that, if I resolv'd to leave without a word, and never see her more, I might carry it off; but, if I had to explain to her, my resolve should-surely collapse

""Whether we might have been happy, living with my shame that I had deserted my master, will never be know'n.

"I need not relate with what sentiments I read in Boswell's 'Life', after the Doctor's passing, his admonition that a person should abstain from making vows, his reason being his profess'd certitude that they are inevitably broken."

"Surely, he must have been referring specifically to Mister Boswell in this."

"I have come to cherish that belief, sir; for a man calls upon belief where he can find no certainty."

CHAPTER SEVEN

IN WHICH SIR JOSHUA REYNOLDS FOUNDS THE LITERARY CLUB,
MASTER FRANCIS SEEKS ADVICE FROM DOCTOR LEVET, AND A
SURPRISE VISITOR ARRIVES AT INNER TEMPLE LANE.

"Our return to London was a cold affair, then, for more reasons than the weather, which lay bleakly indeed, being assisted by an horrible north wind. In despite of our blankets and greatcoats, our fingers became blue and stiff (though The Doctor, as ever, refus'd to acknowledge any inconvenience of an atmospherickal nature). The horses' breath was like smoak upon the air, and their hoof-falls were muffl'd by the frosty ground. Even the coach-springs were stiffen'd by the cold, multiplying the jarring familiar enough in that form of locomotion.

"Well do I remember how my spirits rais'd on passing through Shoreditch and Bishopsgate, when I knew there would soon be a fire and familiar things to close about me, as if the jaunt to Langton never had been.

"Within weeks, while the snow still lay upon the ground, Sir Joshua advanc'd the idea of the Club. Indeed, the thing had been talk'd about for some considerable period of time, but 'twas now put in hand with some expediency, so that it actually came to meet quite soon after our return.

"Its purpose was debate and discussion, the taking of good food and drink in sound company, and, of course, the up-lifting, by association, of its members, one with the other.

"In short, it provided, for one day a week, all those things that Doctor Johnson held most dear; and, for as long as he could attend it, he was at the fulcrum of it. We can make a good wager that he held the floor for the majority of its minutes, though 'twas Sir Joshua who chose its meeting-place, at the Turk's Head, in Gerrard Street, near to his house in Leicester Fields.

"I remember that there were nine original members, though the club has since grown somewhat. I cannot now name all of them, but they included, as well as Sir Joshua and the Doctor, Mister Langton, Mister Beauclerk, Mister Burke, Mister Goldsmith and the Knight.

"Its name is now The Literary Club, Mister Langton and Mister Burke still present; but Mister Sheridan, whom my late Master call'd 'Sherry', is now join'd, with two very fine men: Mister Windham and The Bishop of Dromore, who have been friends to me in this life. Not now among their number is the Knight, who continued to be, as my Master describ'd him: 'a most un-club-able man', being, finally, so rude in his behaviour, that he was ignor'd by the other members, and, taking the inference, came no more.

"The Master and I were still in residence at Inner Temple Lane at that time. The Williams woman was lodg'd separately in Bolt Court; so, but that we often had visiters, the house was very quiet by Johnsonian standards. Doctor Levet was sometimes there, however, though not with any regularity, for the accommodations were limited, and he might sleep with equal comfort in the rookeryes with his patients, as upon a bolster in the garrett.

"Indeed, if some one's end were nigh (as 'twas often among his poor charges), he would base him-self at their bed-side, going about his walk (which was from Houndsditch to Marybone) from there.

"Betimes, he would call upon us for tea, and report upon his doings. If he should be there, Mister Johnson (which is what he was still at that time, though I have acquir'd the habit of using his title) would join us, drinking the lion's share of the tea, and exhibiting no obvious sign that he was listening to anything Doctor Robert had to say.

"This, like his gyrations, and his habit of conversing with himself, was merely a peculiarity of the Master's character. Though he give neither encouragement nor acknowledgement, he would absorb all information imparted to him, adding it to his universal store.

"My own measure of wisdom cannot be as potent as that of my Master, but I have never deny'd a powerfull desire for its augmentation.

"He would often set aside time to instruct and guide me, which was what I valued above all else; so much so, indeed, that I could never ask aught of him, being ever convinc'd that what he did for me was more than I had the right to expect.

"In later years, at the house in Bolt Court, when he would gather the house-hold about him for his 'fire-side chats', he would ask me: 'Why do not you ask me questions?', but I never could take the same liberty with my Master as with another person. Knowledge and wisdom were his especial proficiency; not, therefore, to be lightly taken or given away; whereas an apothecary, a cook, a fisher, or a practitioner of physick, hath knowledge but as a means to the prosecution of his employment, so may share of such information without injury.

"I listen'd with great interest, therefore, to all that Doctor Levet had to relate, more especially when Mister Johnson was abroad; and I had no such hesitation in consulting the full span of his sagacity, which was, by no means, in-considerable.

"Many people never knew aught of him, but that he was rude in his manner. Such people took no interest in him accordingly, but nor did he in them. His interest was in his patients; and they valued him for the quality of his care and his ministrations; not for the graciousness of his deportment.

"So I learnt from him the value of differentiation. True merit requires no puffing-up. Indeed, it may be obscur'd by it. Pritty manners can put a nice polish upon worth; but obsequiousness alone won't do."

"That's sound enough, if not right original."

"My very point to you, sir, is that I was yet young and un-educated. Such ideas to a man who has known nothing but slavery and servitude are original, and, I believe, valued the more for it; for that I was open to learning in a way that most seem not to be.

"I have ever sought to increase my measure of knowledge from all sources; whereas those whose early lives knew not my dis-advantages, attend only to Great Authorityes, and seek only fashionable intelligence; the while failing to observe fundamental truths with-in their own purview.

"Mister Levet was dis-advantag'd in his early years; yet, by his own efforts alone, came to possess enough of knowledge to make him the most usefull man I ever knew. What he had apprehended at a young age in Paris was to change the guiding principle of his life.

"'I am sure that I need to change,' I told him, one morning at Inner Temple Lane.

"'Fie! P'shaw! Change, says you. Well and good, I reply, but from what to what?', he demanded of me, in his characteristick way. 'I would have all my patients well; but first must know in what wise they are ill. The alchymyst would have gold from the transformation of base metal; but is frustrated, for he knoweth not the propertyes of the base-metal, so cannot hope to devyse a method for its transmutation. 'Odd's potions, my fine black friend, mark well the path by which ye came, ere ye venture further, or ye'll change nothing, but that ye be compleatly lost!'

"This was typickal of the manner in which he would instruct me. Leaving me with such a thought to muse upon, he would slam down his tea-cup and be on his way.

"I would go with him to the street-door, and watch him out of sight as he went to make an appearaunce in one of the many other lives, in which he took such a vital part.

"On one such day, as I stood in the door-way, looking after him, I beheld something that brought me up short; indeed, I thought myself struck by madness! I turn'd into the darkness of the interior to clear my eyes; then look'd back again; but the vision remain'd, and, seeing me in return, dropt its valise and ran forward, crying: 'Frank! Frank! I have found you!'"

"What's this? Someone from your past?" I was not a little reliev'd by this turn from philosophy back to incident.

"'Twas none other than that sweet girl I had lately deserted in Lincolnshire, fetch'd up in my London life, to which she no-wise belong'd."

"You don't say so!"

"That I do, sir, right verily."

"What did you do?"

"I gogg'd, sir, like an ideot; and I ran about in my head, looking for a thought, or an idea, that might do some service; but I found nothing there.

"Then, fortunately, some one try'd to make off with her valise, which was something I could answer, so I broke away from her, and ran and knock'd him down; laying about him and a-pulling of his hair, while I might gather myself to decide what should be done with the girl.

"But I might have tore every hair from off the culprit's scurvy head, and still be none the wiser, so I ran him into Fleet Street, and return'd to the cause of my confusion."

"She must have lov'd you greatly to have undertaken such a pursuit! How came she there?" I must own that I was not entirely convinc'd that this wasn't a sailor's tale or a romantick fiction, for the girl must have travell'd near two hundred miles - a long step for a rural lass - with naught at the end but finding a black servant in a place the size of London. To say it was an unlikely thing, would not be unjust, to be sure.

"I embrac'd her, though I could summon little of the warmth I had felt in Lincolnshire, and led her to the kitchen. I could not respond in a suitable way to the situation, because I knew not how I should respond.

"Nothing in my experience had prepar'd me for it. All I could think of was that she shouldn't be there - in the Master's house. She was out of place; aye, and out of time.

"Mister Johnson had as much as order'd me to forget her, and that I had; the taking of orders being what I did.

"Whereas in Lincolnshire, it had been all un-reasoning emotion and infatuation; in London I saw everything against it. Her presence endanger'd all that I had; and all that I would have. 'Twas selfishness, I admit, but I had much chang'd since we had our idyll in the country. I had begun to form a notion of what I wanted; and she was not connected with it.

"She was sweet; she was loving; she was brave; she was pritty; aye, and she was intelligent; but she was no more than a sweet, loving, brave, pritty, and intelligent problem; and I could not suppress the idea that, if the Master thought her presence any of my doing, he would cast me out with her.

"She look'd as out of place in that kitchen as a nun in a ship's galley: 'Art thou pleas'd to see me, Franky?' says she. Well, I could neither tell her a lye nor the truth, as you will readily see. 'Sit thee down,' says I, 'Thou must be greatly fatigu'd from thy journey.' 'Ah, no,' says she, 'I've not come far today, for I journey'd with the drovers, and have been a-while at Epping; but, the prices now being right, we mov'd on to London yesterday, and I am come this morning from Smithfield.'

"The kettle was still simmering over the fire from Doctor Levet's parting, so I made her some tea, while I thought out the best way to deal with her. At least, she had not travell'd alone from Lincolnshire (as I, at first, fear'd), so might, likewise, be able to catch up with the drovers for the return.

"I decided how I could best serve my own advantage. 'I was about to go on an errand upon thy arrival,' I said. 'Rest thee there, and take what thou wilt of tea and bread, 'till I return to thee anon.'

"Then I set off in search of the Master, that I could tell him what had come to pass and, in so doing, absolve myself from any cause, so he would put her right; but not put me wrong in the doing thereof, if you take my meaning!"

"You were not very kind, Master Barber, that you did not tell her your true feelings, in a manly fashion, and be done."

"Kind, sir? No, sir. Nor was I. Indeed, I had never before had anyone to be kind to, and had not the art of it.

"Some had been kind to me; others less so. I had been grateful, un-grateful, obedient and dis-obedient. No, sir; I had not been kind."

"Did you know where your Master was to be found?"

"No, but 'twas never too great a difficultye finding him, for he was remarkable enough in his appearaunce; without he progress'd in such a singular fashion that he could not but draw attention to himself.

"He went everywhere with a very large stick, with which he would tap each tethering post along the way, a-counting to himself as he went. He had by heart the number of some of these posts from frequent use - those at crossings, or at the entrances to yards and courts - so if he should mis-count, he would return to one such before continuing to tap along his way.

"He kept his left hand all-ways to his chest, except when, for reasons no one was ever able to fathom, he would stop dead and commence upon one of his gyrations; following which, he often abandon'd his original course and, either embark'd upon a new, or return'd whence he had come.

"For these reasons, he rarely pass'd un-notic'd, and, on that morning, had been observ'd by many, heading for the Turk's Head Coffee House in the Strand, where he often went, saying: 'I encourage this house, for the mistress of it is a good civil woman, and has not much business.'

"I found him there, and convey'd the substaunce of the difficulty to him. He told me that I must repair to Inner Temple Lane, and see about her entertainment until he should return; and that I should, in no way, encourage her affections or misunderstandings in the meanwhile.

"I told him that this should prove difficult for me, for that I did not wish to hurt her; to which he reply'd: 'You will hurt her the more, if you use her love when you have not a right to it. Be truthful in this, Frank,' said he, 'and it will ameliorate significantly your future relations.'.

"My reason and experience told me he was right in this, though my heart wanted conviction. I return'd to the house, but the walk back was long, and my feet heavy

"My primary impulse was to avoid the problem; to go off into the alley-ways until it be all over and done with.

"I had no taste for responsibility, and no aptitude for it. My mentality was that of the slave: keep yourself unto yourself, and do as you are told, until you can run away.

"To run away was the dream of all of my brothers and sisters in Jamaica."

"'Tis, by no means, confin'd to them, you can be sure."

"Nay, so I have come to learn. It remain'd my early impulse. All activity was the responsibility of, and impos'd upon us by, another, whom we must serve; hence, we sought escape from service, and crav'd in-activity. Certain among us were eventually to find both."

"Quite so!" I laugh'd at this ironickal reference to his present life (as I took it to be).

"No other person than the Master could have caus'd me to overturn my instincts. He was the root of any certainty, and my vow was as a rock. I must do as he told me, even were it to bring me harm, which I knew it would not in the fullness of time.

"But, for all I was cowardly for my own part, I was also concern'd for her; for 'twas I that had changed, not she. She had been constant to the Francis she had met in Lincolnshire, but had arriv'd to be met with the London Francis, which she did not know, and would not find so love-able.

"I summon'd such courage as I had, and enter'd the house. Before that I came to the kitchen, I could hear that she was crying. 'Be still,' I told her, as gently as I was able, 'I'm not worthy of thy tears. I had not thought to trifle with thee. Thou art the only girl I have ever lov'd, but I cannot give thee what I have not to give. My life is not yet mine own, and may never be. I will not put thee through whate'er it hold, for it might break thee, and, so doing, break me too. Go back safe to thy home, and find there some one to cherish thee as thou shou'd'st be cherish'd. My love for thee wisheth for the best that life can give thee, which I, in no wise, am, for I am not yet become my own man, which I must be ere I can consent or hope to be another's'.

"I knew not where the words had come from, nor the strength to say them, but they touch'd her, and she left off crying, though her breathing was short.

"A-drying of her tears with her apron, she drew herself up, so that I was reminded of the pride and bearing that had stolen my senses at Langton: 'I know not what ideas thou may'st have form'd, sir, but I think that thou mistaketh me; for I had merely thought to visit mine especial friend, with whom I had enjoy'd a brief amour, to tell him, that he will be ever after remember'd, warmly and affectionately, as the one who taught me how to love.'

"Now I was the one in tears, for she had more strength of character than I might ever have, and 'twould have been an easy thing to fall in love with her, over again. Though I could barely speak, I said: 'And I shall ever hold thee the same, for I might never have known what love was, far less that it might have any connexion to me. Thou hast open'd my soul to the possibility of its improuvement, and my life to hope.'

"We kiss'd as friends, though lingeringly, as if to seal our memoryes, and she said she would now return to her travelling companions, who would be sleeping that night upon the bulks at Smithfield, for an early start upon the morrow.

"I insisted that I should carry her valise thither, and accompany her safely through the mean streets of the Capital, to which she agreed, inasmuch as we should part before she came up with her friends.

"So we set off along Fleet Street and through the Old Bailey. We walk'd separate at first, our faces grim and our foot-steps heavy; but, of a sudden, she link'd my arm and smiled; and, me doing likewise, we went on lightly, 'till we were almost a-skipping; by-standers shouting to us, and we shouting back; until we was come to Smithfield, where, in a flourish, I gave her her valise, and she danc'd away; so we were parted ere the melancholy could return!

"I knew she would get over it now; and, knowing that, so could I."

"A most affecting tale; but were you not already 'over it' ere she arriv'd?"

"I'll take a turn with the cyder flagon, by your leave, Master Reporter, lest an excess of it should have a disagreeable effect upon you.

"It had not been as easy as you might imagine to push her from my mind at the conclusion of the Lincolnshire jaunt, and that is all I had done. She was still there, but had been order'd out. Now I might verily say that I would get over her."

"Pish, sir. No offence meant. 'Twas only a rag."Master

Barber was more accurate than I cared to admit. The cyder, being an un-familiar beverage, had taken me somewhat un-awares, so that my disposition was in danger of alteration. "What said old Johnson, if aught?"

"'Well, now, Frank, my boy, let's have a look at your hay-maker. Where's she hid?'.

"'She is gone, Master, and the matter satisfactorily concluded.'

"He stood before me, in his dear rolling way, staring at me for some time, as if reading my mind. Then he kiss'd me on the forehead, saying: 'Ten years since, Doctor Bathurst told you of the gift of your freedom. Today, you loos'd its wrappings.'.

"I felt a great inner power as I comprehended what he was saying.

"Then he made us kneel: 'Let us pray.'"

CHAPTER EIGHT

IN WHICH THERE IS A MOVE TO JOHNSON'S COURT; THE
THRALES COME UPON THE SCENE AND MASTER BARBER
PHILOSOPHIZES ON THE ADVANCEMENT OF TRADESPEOPLE
AND SERVANTS

"The following year, the Master finally completed his *Shakespeare.* What with his pension and some money from reviews, he was now financially improuv'd, but the material for his *Shakespeare* was all over the place at Temple Lane, so he could not think to leave that house until he had done.

"Once it was off to the printers, he set in train the re-assemblage of the house-hold, and found a big enough house in Johnson's Court, which was back across Fleet Street again; near to Gough Square, and to Bolt Court, where Mrs. Williams lodg'd.

"I assisted the carter in the removal, which was a piece-meal affair, since no packing-up had been done; so we would have cooking pots, books, and cloaths, all upon the cart together; and many things were never seen more.

"Because of we had neither boxes nor crates, all the chattels and paraphernalia was strewn about in no particular order, and arriv'd at the other end likewise.

"The only things which came to the house in an organised way were those of Mrs. Williams, who now mov'd with us into the new house. 'Tis true that I often speak ill of her, for we were of violently opposing characters, and could no-wise get along in each other's companye. But, the manner in which she coped with her affliction was a wonder to all who knew her.

"She was stone-blind, yet she had pack'd her belongings meticulously, so that they were properly sorted, and protected from harm upon the cart. What's more, she knew where every item had been pack'd, and could lay her hands upon't directly.

"For all that she could be ill-humour'd and ambagious in her speech, I believe she lov'd the Master greatly; and, though she had not the greatest ease herself, she was ever about good deeds and charitable doings for those with less."

"How did she maintain herself?"

"She receiv'd of a number of small allowances from different sources, I believe; none of which would have kept her for long, but she manag'd upon the sum of them.

"The one thing, other than love of the Master, that we had in common was our partiality for neatness and order (though my cause was lost in the matter of the Master's possessions). She was very particular about the keeping of her belongings and affairs, so liv'd tolerable well, in her way.

"Also, she publish'd poetry; sometimes of her own writing, other times collected from other poets. The Master was very solicitous of her in this, and assisted in every way he could, including the writing of something for her to put in a book, which, I should think, help'd to sell it. When they were together, he call'd her Jenny.

"Doctor Levet also came back to live with us, now we had space for him, though, of course, he had no effects, but for his medical box.

"This had been good for the Master, for he had been oppress'd with the melancholy while at Inner Temple Lane, but came to himself right quickly when he had the in-mates once more about him.

"Also, at this time, he heard that the University of Dublin had made him into a Doctor of Laws, which both surpriz'd and pleas'd him greatly, he having wanted a degree, but given up the thought of getting one.

"But neither the move nor the degree wrought the biggest change that was to come in that year. A new chapter was to begin for us all by his acquaintaunce with Mister and Mistress Thrale of Streatham."

"He was a brewer, wasn't he? And she went on to be Mrs. Piozzi?"

"Correct in both particulars, sir.

"Mister Henry Thrale was one of those men of our time, who, having come forth from humble beginnings, make of themselves a figure in the world, acquiring such merit and such manners as fit them for the companye, aye, and the respect of the quality.

"His father had been an employee of the brewery, when the woman who would have inherited it marry'd a nobleman, who had no interest in its continuation. Old Mister Thrale persuaded the woman's aged parent to make the concern over to him, whereafter he improuv'd the business to such a degree that he was able to pay off the price of it with-in eleven years.

"Being a prudent, as well as a capable man, he profited well in his trade, and put much of the money to the bringing on of his son, who was given the best of educations, and sent upon the Grand Tour, like a gentleman.

"For those reasons, Henry came to be very refin'd, with tastes much above his birth, and a fine house, which he builded in the country south of London at Streatham Park. There would gather many of the luminaryes of those years, and the Master would find it a most agreeable place away from his beloved London to spend time in contemplation, in perusing the excellent library, and in the grand company which there assembl'd.

"Mister Henry's wyfe, Hester, was bright and quick. She was ever a match for conversation, and had a love of art and wit, which made her a favourite in the Doctor's life for many years.

"I was sorry when he took against her marriage to Signor Piozzi, for it turn'd an happy association sour at the end. He could not accept that she was enough her own person to choose wisely in the matter of a successor to Mister Henry.

"Also, it is my belief that the Master shou'd have marry'd her himself."

"What? Johnson and Mrs. Thrale wed? I know naught of such a proposition." The un-happy effect of the Lichfield cyder upon my humour and my speech had now begun to diminish, so that I could reclaim my place at this inter-view with a little more vigour than of late.

"Nay, sir. I'm sure you do not, for the degree of intimacy between Doctor Johnson and Mrs. Thrale was not suspected by

Mister Boswell or the Knight, and has been obscur'd in the lady's own accounts.

"What are you suggesting, Master Barber? I hope you do not intend to besmirch thy Master's reputation; or that of the lady." As a journalist, I have no taste for scandal, as you may be sure.

"Suggesting, sir? I, sir? Nothing, sir; but nor will I give you a false or prittify'd idea of people who were as good as they were, on the one side; and only as bad as they were, upon the other. As I said before, we need only screen those who are unfit to be clearly seen. I do not believe either to be deserving of that description."

"Well and good; well and good. Explain, then, to what intimacy you are referring."

"That I will, sir, but at its proper time.

"These were the early days of their acquaintaunce, when it was a simple burgeoning of friend-ship that was a-taking place. She was a very direct person; a jolly sort, and she enliven'd the Master greatly, when he could easily become prey to the horrours.

"Mister Thrale was as severe as she was jovial, giving no quarter in his dealings with the house-hold, nor with the trades-men neither. Some on his servants was much against him, saying he was un-pleasaunt and abrupt, but I found him honest and fair; and he gave, every year, an entertainment for the house-hold, and any of their friends, family, and, even, on occasion, lovers, as they might like to invite, which was generously done.

"Most of the problem they had with him deriv'd from his not having been 'born to it', as the saying is. I've no doubt but that it can be hard for a man to take command of servants when he's had no bringing-up in that direction. I know for a fact that it is un-natural to receive orders from such a man; many people in service no-wise able to come used to it."

"So, it is true, in your view, that some are born to give, and others to take orders."

"I believe that to be the way of it, commonly; yes, sir. I do not believe there to be any reason, other than precedent, for such an arrangement, except inasmuch as for every thing that some one can make or do, there must be another in need. In order for the person who can make or do a thing to live by it, there must be a proportionate number of people a-wanting of it.

"Our time is changing, as Mister Thrale himself was proof of. He was a servant to those who look'd for fine ale, but he was a master to his house-hold. Some traditional divisions are much alter'd by the urban-isation of society, which we have seen in London; but you will not yet find it to the same degree here at Lichfield, and it has not begun at Tor Bay.

"The trades-people are a better class of servant, and they are coming up all the time.

"I was born a slave, but my first master made me into a freed man, and my second into a man of property. You have heard that the Colonel's declaration had no material effect upon my person; and you shall later hear (if there be time, and your interest persists) how I have fared in Doctor Johnson's design."

"Don't doubt that I would hear all you have to tell me, should it take all night in the telling,"I told him, though the day was advancing apace.

He said nothing to this, but continued his thought: "It could be said, and is said in his servants' hall, that Mister Thrale was born to be a journeyman brewer. His father made him proprietor of the brewery, Oxford made of him a scholar, and his fortune made him master at Streatham Park; but nothing could make of him a gentleman in the eyes of those of his own class and below; likely in his own eyes neither."

"The accident of birth is all then; and change is impossible."

"Impossible? No, sir. It is possible, but it is no easy under-taking."

He was pensive again. "Not easy at all, sir."

"Yet the Thrales seem to have found no difficulty in being accepted by polite society."

"Ah, Polite is the word, sir. The society of those with the politesse and the imagination to stretch a point, sir; those who could afford to allow the transformation; and those who believ'd such a transformation the worthiest of all ambitions; which was not necessarily the view of others, if you take my meaning.

"In that, Mister Thrale was not so different from Doctor Johnson, whose father was a provincial book-seller, it should be remembered. He was adopted by society for his accomplishments, his wisdom and his diversionary value. The Thrales gather'd at their house such as he to attract those with whom they would be associated, so that they were all elevated in their different fashions.

"That first year, the Doctor was to stay at Streatham from July to September; a long period for him to stay away from London. It was too long for me, so I soon acquir'd the habit of walking between the Park and Johnson's Court."

"That's a fair walk, is it not?"

"Nay, sir; half a dozen miles, and good roads all the way. 'Tis no more than might be walk'd in a day's commerce, and thought nothing of. I have walk'd two miles today, since receiving of your summons."

CHAPTER NINE

IN WHICH YOUR REPORTER ATTEMPTS TO DEFINE THE
RELATIONSHIP BETWEEN MASTER BARBER AND THE DOCTOR,
AND THE FORMER TALKS OF EDUCATION (HIS OWN AND THAT
OF THE LOCAL YOUTH)

I had not been in Master Barber's company above four hours, but it is interesting to reflect to what degree my perception of him had chang'd in that time.

Though it is all-ways my endeavour to avoid the formation of pre-conceptions in such a case, a certain measure of these inevitably enters in, as a result of that preparation, in the form of study and research, which must be done ere an inter-view or report is undertaken.

In this particular case, such preparation was, of necessity, limited, there being no comprehensive record of the subject's life and doings upon which to draw. Indeed, almost the only matter consists of peripheral references in works having Johnson at their centre.

Though there be such a paucity of material, a universal image of the man has been receiv'd; and, probably because there is so little information, that image is easily disseminated.

Before making his acquaintaunce, I had a clear idea of what I expected. He would be black. He would be humble. He would be simple. He would be comfortably off. He would be a bit of a peacock as to dress and personal adornment. He would speak in only reverential and subdued terms about his master and those of the quality. He would be all gratitude; and he would be soon done with.

When tested against the reality, but one of these propositions stood up.

The faithful negro servant was a myth, born, like so many such, from incomplete observation.

He seem'd to be trying to tell me something about the nature of a life subject to such pre-conceptions (or were they better call'd mis-conceptions?).

Before the death of Colonel Bathurst, he had been a slave; but that is not all he was. After the colonel's death, he was a freed man; yet he was as much a slave as he had been before; and still he was neither.

Such record as has been printed of his existence exclusively categorises him as Doctor Johnson's servant. A summary perusal of the facts brings us to doubt it.

It seems it was out of his power to render himself very useful as a servant, yet the Doctor would not cast him off on that account; and, when the master was no more, he provided a staff to support him in his stead.

So the best we can do is to describe him as Johnson's companion; but he could not be such at table, at the Literary Club, or at the levées of Johnson's friends; and was not such on the jaunts to the Western Isles, to Wales or to France.

We might almost be better, then, to say Johnson's protégé but, if that be so, for what did his patron fit him? We have it from Barber's own account that he is not the toast of local society, and we can see how 'twould be so.

There was more yet to be got to the bottom of; not least the import of certain ominous sayings of his, earlier in the day. And, while I continued to be interested in my original mission of getting another view-point of the Doctor (including the hinted-at revelations concerning that party and Mrs. Thrale, to be sure!), I would know more of Francis Barber for his own sake.

The cyder was now finish'd - a circumstance I was, by no means, regretful of - so I consulted him as to his disposition toward the continuation of our walk. He reply'd that he was more than ready, and that, if we were to return the flagon to the farm, we might continue in that way to come out by Stow-hill, which suited me right well, the house there being on my list of Johnsonian sites.

The common gave way to hedges and stone-walls as we continued our climb, and we came soon to Scott's Farm, whence my companion had fetch'd the cyder, before proceeding to the rocky ridge, and descending into Stow-hill-lane, from where we could get a fair view of Miss Aston's house, at which Johnson had more than once been a guest.

At the foot of the lane is, perhaps, the most picturesque place in Lichfield, for here is to be found St. Chad's Church, the Barber family's regular place of worship. This is a minor parish church of great beautye, in as near perfect a setting as could be imagin'd.

Next the church, across a water-logg'd lane, is Stow-mill, which is also most pleasing and quaint, with its flotillas of playful water-fowls. The real glory of the scene, though, is the prospect it affords across Stowe-water to the towne; a panorama from the heights to the left, across the roofes of Stow-street, with the tower of St. Mary's standing proud, to the houses of the Quonians and the sublime Minster, with their perfect inverse reflections in the water, upon the right hand.

Un-willing to quit this tranquille place until it should be necessary, we found new resting-places, our backs to the trunks of two trees that o'erhang the waterside track; plac'd so that we might watch the day mature upon this noble prospect.

We had chatted about this and that, while walking thither. Master Barber was keen about his fishing, which he did with a rod, formerly the property of Johnson, and much coveted by his fellow-fishers. It not being a subject of which I possess any degree of skill or knowledge, I must ask your comprehension of my inability to record details of his method, and the types of fish which predominate in the Pool, both of which he favour'd me with, but neither of which I have retain'd, finding in my mind, in their stead, the celebrated Johnsonian description of angling: 'A stick and a string, with a worm at one end, and a fool at the other.'

It came to me to wonder why he had chosen to remove to Lichfield on his Master's death. Why, for example, had he not chosen to go to Devon, where he had been much taken with the scenery? He again grew mysterious on this point, but told me how he had first come to the place with Johnson near the end of his life, when they had also gone to Ashbourne, Birmingham and Oxford.

"It was but a month before his passing that we were in this place; and it was fitting, though he no more felt at home, and was distrest at the change; which must happen to a man who hath such memoryes of his growing up, and trys to return at last. I believe I have come closer to his home than he was. But I think that my design is clearer," he told me, though he would not be prest to explain his final remark.

As we settled ourselves by the Pool, he confided that he had a fancy to teach school. I must confess that I did not take him seriously on this point, it requiring too great an exercise of imagination.

"Why should you find such a proposition so surprising, sir? Both my wyfe and myself are possess'd of a level of education far above the general run of people hereabouts.

"We have children of our own, whom we have brought up and taught ourselves; and it is my feeling that the greatest legacy of the Doctor was not his money, but the fact that he educated me sufficiently to contemplate the appropriation of my own life.

"He oft express'd a desire to run a school him-self; indeed, he did so for a period, near here at Ediall, though he had not enough of maturity nor authority to succeed at that early period of his life

"I would do with such as remains of his legacy what I can to prosecute his own wishes. Though his money and possessions be made over to me, still they are his. I have them in trust, for I did not earn them.

"My parts do not fit me for literary endeavour; nor to be the witty darling of the Quality. But there is no reason, of which I am aware, that prevents me from imparting knowledge and training to the children of the trades-people and labourers.

"The Doctor saw to it that my own education was sound and comprehensive, not merely in the stuff of normal schooling, such as reading and writing, but in the disciplines of reason and perception, of which he was the greatest master.

"I can teach no one mathematicks or the management of money; but I might teach them how to express themselves; and

I might expand their capacity for learning, that they might, like me, see beyond the identityes placed upon them by ignorance and habit, and follow the Lord, Jesus Christ's injunction: Know thyself; for, from the highest to the lowest, though you have the prittiest store of learning and studye conceivable, if you know not your self, you know naught." He convey'd this sentiment with a passion not far remov'd from violence.

The longer I remain'd in his companye, the plainer became the explanation for his dis-connexion from the fashionable world. Though he be of low birth, he is such that might have been well-receiv'd at all the best tables, for his nouveauté, as well as for his Johnsonian value. His manners are entirely acceptable, as to speech and deportment, but that his address is too forthright and his opinions are too forcefully exprest, which was tolerated, or even fêted, in Johnson, but would, in no wise, be acceptable from an elevated lacquey.

The degree of that elevation continued to astonish me. He could discourse (at great length, you may be sure) upon subjects which remain closed to some who have had all the benefices of breeding and instruction society can offer. I am prepared to own that I had more than a little difficulty in following certain of his conceptions until long after this meeting.

There was in him a species of natural clarity, and sharpness of perception, which enabled him to see through what his master call'd *cant*; yet he manag'd his life like an on-looker, being ever able to accurately chronicle it, though seeming powerless to direct it.

I made this last observation to him.

"Is a servant not expected to carry out instructions with precision, sir? In order so to do, must he not have complete understanding of what is expected of him? Or, if he have not, must he not speedily acquire such understanding? A servant hath not the liberty to abandon a topick that o'erstretches him, sir. He must master it; and he need not trouble to report upon the difficulty with which such mastery was obtain'd; that is the leisure activity of a dabbler or a dilettante.

"As to your saying that I seem powerless in the direction of my life, sir, I take it not amiss, for it is a business I am but lately come into.

"If I may call myself a man in all other things, yet I am a callow adolescent in this enterprise, but I advance apace.

"In due time, the pupil must become the teacher; the servant, the master."

I recall'd reading that he had completed his own schooling in Northamptonshire, so inquir'd as to that.

"'Twas not Northamptonshire, sir. I know not the origin of that idea; though 'tis but another instaunce of transformation, of that kind with which I am ever troubled."

"An insignificant failing of research or memory, to be sure; naught more perturbaceous than that!" It were passing trivial, to my mind.

"An insignificant thing, indeed, sir, that dis-lodges a man in time and space! No cause for alarum in that!"

"Hold, Master Barber! Boswell was not idle, though the woman on the stage-coach may have thought him so; you were not at school in Northamptonshire, though I may have thought so. What of it?"

"There is material evidence (in the shape of his literary works) to prove that Boswell was not idle. No evidence exists that I was in Bishop Stortford, rather than Northamptonshire, other than that someone should say so.

"'Tis hard enough for a man to take back a life that has been o'er-ruled, without it be liable to posterior travesty!"

I conceded his point, contrary though I then thought it to be. "'Twas Bishop Stortford, then; Hertfordshire, if I'm not mistaken."

"Exactly so, sir. Bishop Stortford Grammar School, to be precise. Upon the road to Cambridge - and as far down the same as I am ever like to travel, as you might say.

"The school there was founded by a man call'd Clapp, with whose widow Doctor Johnson lodg'd me for the duration.

"With Old Mister Clapp's demise had come a crisis in the school funds, so that, when I was come there, in the Spring following, all was disorder, and became steadily worse.

"The Reverend Mister Fowler had been appointed to Head Master ere the truth of the financial situation came to light, so that he was a victim of the circumstaunce, a-like to the rest on us.

"I must own to a certain ironick humour at the eventuality that the school to which the Master chose to send me should prove as paradoxickal as himself!

"I wrote him a number of letters, informing him of the irregularityes, and seeking his advice; but his experience led him to expect perplexity, so he bade me hold my ground, which pay'd off at last, and I remain'd there a full four years, finding the Reverend a most effectual teacher, and his masters likewise (Mister Ellis and Mister Smith).

"It must be reported, however, that it was not all-ways a simple matter to attend to the lessons, since the house in which the school was quarter'd, stood upon pillars atop the Market Place.

"No, sir. Not for us the hallow'd hush of academe. Bishop Stortford's was a most vociferous method of education, sir.

"By the time I had stay'd there two years, with ne'er a visit, I began to form the belief that I had been abandon'd there, and I wrote to the Doctor to tell him so. I don't know if he had forgot me, for he had been in poor health; but he sent me a letter that restor'd my determination to succeed, in which he said: 'Do not imagine that I shall forget or forsake you; for if, when I examine you, I find that you have not lost your time, you shall want no encouragement', to which he was all-ways true.

"I later made a copy of this letter and sent it to Mister Boswell, for it was, to me, a precious record of his true sentiments."

CHAPTER TEN

IN WHICH FURTHER EFFORTS ARE MADE TO ASCERTAIN THE EXACT FORM OF THE RELATIONSHIP BETWEEN MASTER AND SERVANT

Johnson must have been convinced of the merit, and capacity for learning of, his Francis, to be sure, for he spent more than three hundred pounds upon his education.

We can also deduce, with some certainty, that his purpose was altruistick; since education of this sort is unlikely to produce a better servant (indeed, rather the contrary), and, for the duration of the said education, he was depriv'd of both service and companion-ship.

Could it be, perhaps, that there was some ultimate design in the thing? Did he have it in his mind to make of Francis an amanuensis or copyist?

"No, sir. He never gave me any copying, or any writing down to do that was not an exercise-toward its intrinsick perfection

"He kept me applyd to such exercises, and would not permit of a single day's lapse in them, while he was there to see to it. When he was away, he would set me a syllabus, and charge Mister Levet (or, other-wise Mrs. Williams) with the super-vision."

"So it would seem that he regarded your improuvement as an end of itself. Yet, you must have been approaching thirty years of age; did you not feel rebellious at being super-vised thus, as a child?"

"No, sir. At least, not upon the whole; for, the more I apprehended, the more I valued the learning, coming to see how it applyd to mine own case. Taken together, it is clear that there were no other end to the Doctor's learning than its own increase.

"He oft pointed out that the simplest book which is now written would be an un-imaginable undertaking, did it not draw upon the learnings and the codifications of vaste numbers of antecedents.

"Though it be thought that an individual man's sagacity die with him, yet he may have contributed something to that store of common-knowledge which advances the cause of society and mankind in general. That is the inference I drew from his many utterances upon the subject. He believ'd nothing to be more valuable than the increase of knowledge, and I am certainly of his opinion.

"But, like him also, I am now come to conclude that wisdom will not gain ascendancy through Occultation; so that I intend, as previously said, to pass on such of mine as I might to the children hereabout.

"While I was so taken up in its acquiring, I had no thoughts as to its purpose or final end. Whether the Doctor ever thought upon the outcome will never be know'n (though I'll wager he did); but, with what-ever clarity he might have descryd it, we may be certain that he would have continued upon his course.

"In accordaunce with his belief, he would consult the learning of others, choosing to accept or reject its conclusions with reference to his own experience. Once accepting of it, it were as it had been his own idea from the first, so that he would deliver it with absolute conviction, and want no support from its original authour.

"Those ideas which were of his origination proceeded all-ways from his own experience or experiment. He would oftentimes set in train processes of essay, probation and verification, embracing physick, chymystry, human constitution and natural philosophy.

"I must use these terms to express to you the wide range of his interest, though he was not happy with the categorization of knowledge, which cannot but be a limiter thereof. Any thing which affects, or relates to, mankind, comes with-in the domain of its knowledge. Each man, if he would truly he a man, should be in constant quest of greater knowledge - of himself, his fellowes, the world, and his chosen (or necessitous) sphere of endeavour. He that is not, would live out his life as a brute; and the Doctor would have him treated as one!

"Learning, then, was not (is not) an activity to be confin'd to youth. Those who study in their later years have no need to feel childish. They may, indeed, feel somewhat superior to those around them, who are not studying; as I did.

"Also, at that time, I was entrusted with the provisioning of the house-hold and the budgeting for same, which was not a task to set a child upon."

Again, he spoke sooth in this.

Johnson was a man who gather'd dependents about him, by all accounts. As well as his regular in-mates, he was, by no means, averse to taking in waifs and strays which he found in bad state upon the streets.

The regular in-mates seem'd assured of a lodging in perpetuity, for as long as the Master was there to grant it. In a similar way, he supported friends, more or less distant relations, and ex-colleagues when in want, and, in some cases, beyond his own grave.

The street-people who receiv'd of his protection, he re-stored and re-fitted to assume, once more, the life of the street; to which he, himself, was no stranger.

But, in all these cases, it was maintainaunce or repair that were the end of his ministrations.

Only in himself, and in one other, did he expect, or encourage, actual betterment. That other was our present Subject; that person who was also to be the major beneficiary under his Will. We must be satisfied upon this point, ere we can move on. Johnson's motive was not to produce a better servant; it was not to procure an amanuensis; it was not for any specify'd future end.

What about this, then? We hear from all of his acquaintaunce that the Doctor could not abide solitude. Everything he valued in the world had to do with erudite companye.

There would ever be times when, for one reason or another, such companye was either not available, or-not biddable. Is it possible he was trying to make of Francis a companion, not merely in the sense of some one present, but a true adjuvant, able to hold his own, and provide stimulating converse, where none other was to be had?

Our fashionable society being as it is, he might well have anticipated a time in which he should survive its good opinion, and be condemn'd to fall back upon such a provision.

Also, he was not greatly favour'd in the matter of health, and could have become house-bound or, even bed-ridden, in either of which a companion able to read to him, record his thoughts, and talk upon higher things were much to be wish'd for.

"He wanted you for an erudite and stimulating companion, to attend upon him in the absence of society," I announced. "What say you to that proposition, Master Francis?"

"I say, sir, that it is wide of the mark.

"In his company, I kept such erudition as I may have possess'd to myself. I hope I may, on occasion, have been stimulating as a companion; but not of conversation in the sense that you suggest.

"Our companion-ship was of a simple and innocent kind; more akin to a father and his son, sir."

"Aha! Then we are come to it!" Of course, Johnson was deny'd children. His beloved Tetty was already the mother of Miss Lucy Porter ere they were marry'd, and was some twenty years older than he. Although speculations arose concerning a number of possible new wyves in the years after her death, naught came of any of them.

Was Francis (who was, in any case, a likely subject for the Doctor's affections immediately following Tetty's loss - Doctor Bathurst's reasoning when persuading Johnson to take the boy in) a substitute son?

If 'twere the case, it would explain Johnson's patience and solicitude; his desire for the boy to do well and make a good education; and the legacy at last. Yes, it fits in all particulars. "He took you for the son he never had."

"As to that, sir, I won't deny that there may be something in it, for I lov'd him as a father, and no mis-take; but I did not feel as a son to him. I did not feel that he treated me as I believ'd a son would be treated.

"It is likely that, in this, as in so much else, I am un-qualifyd to give an opinion, for I have not known what it should be like to have a father; but I do feel that, were I his son, it would have been other-wise

"He payd much attention to the children of Mrs. Thrale, especially Queenie, whom he playd with often, and clearly lov'd. For all that he was insistent upon her learning and behaviour, he was never as he was with me.

"He had a genuine affection for me, as we have discuss'd, and we were surely friends of the truest sort, but I had not been back from school but a year, when he went to Scotchland with Mister Boswell, leaving me behind. Hardly was he back from that jaunt than he travell'd with Mister and Mrs. Thrale to Lichfield; again, leaving me behind, so that I could not see the town of his birth.

"Was this a father, who did not take his son home? I think not, sir."

"What do you think was in his mind, then?" I ask'd him.

"In all honesty, sir, I believe him to have had two reasons for his actions; two distinct purposes to serve; the one taking nothing from the other.

"I think you are right to persist in your feeling that he was not completely without interest, but I am also certain that he was ever sensible of my interest.

"He lov'd me very much (as a son, if you will), so that he wanted me to come fully to myself; to have the capacity for independaunce; to be elevated in character and in learning, and to achieve self-respect.

"At the same time, however, I was but one of his experiments: to discover what might be made of a poor African rudely trans-planted into an alien milieu.

"In short, then, sir, I had been slave, I was known as servant, I have been call'd companion, and you have suggested son.

"If all of these possess elements of truth, which I'll accept they do, still they are not the whole truth; which is that I was Doctor Johnson's creature."

CHAPTER ELEVEN

IN WHICH MASTER BARBER'S WIFE IS SPOKEN OF AND THE DOCTOR SUFFERS GREAT AFFLICTION

We sat in silence for I know not how long; the timelessness of that halcyon place broken only by the faint rippling of the water, and the creeping of the shadows, as the sun commenced its descent toward the western hills.

At the far end of the Pool, next the Minster, young couples and knots of townes-people began to appear upon the Reeves' Path (a track skirting the northern shore) for their twilight promenade.

"You mention'd your wyfe, Master Francis. I believe she is a white woman."

"I believe so, too, sir."

"You suggested that she is well-educated, and as fitted for teaching school as yourself. I know that you have been marryd about seventeen years, that she is call'd Elizabeth, and that Mrs. Thrale has described her as 'eminently pretty'; but that is all I know."

"Seventeen years, you say. I dare say you are right upon that point. Well, there's a life for you! Not much to it; swiftly dealt with! But, of course, you humour me, for, if you are cognizant of Mrs. Thrale's 'eminently pretty', you must also be familiar with her 'violently jealous'."

"I own I may have heard, or read, something of the sort. I assume you had your reasons."

"Reasons; yes, sir. A man all-ways has reasons; and, if his actions be a little strange, and his temper seem out of order, we would do well to look to his reasons."

He did not seem dispos'd to continue upon the topick; but, at the risk of giving offense, I tryd a gentle inquiry: "In its early days, it is clear that your marriage did not go easy. Do you believe that you had cause to be jealous, Master Francis?"

"There is ever a cause, sir. The question is, rather, did the cause possess its own independent existence, or was it self-inflicted? No easy question to answer, I must tell you.

"'Eminently pretty', said Mrs. Thrale, and she did not o'erstate it. Beautiful is what she was, sir; and still is; not just in my eyes neither.

"She could have had any man she wanted. Not only was she beautiful; she was clever, too. She had a quick mind, was good in the way of reading and writing, and had taken the trouble to improuve her understanding of the world through books.

"As I have already told you, I had had little to do with love, and thought it a mysterious and slippery thing, not to be trusted; the only time I had been touch'd by it before being the fugitive affair with the hay-maker.

"Why, then, should some one as cultured and desirable as Elizabeth bother with the likes of me? None could explain it to me in such a fashion as I could accept of it, least of all she!

"I could not believe but that there was some delusion; some trick attached to it. I could only think that an elabourate comedy was being play'd out, with me as its fool. I could not leave her in other companye without I thought they were laughing at my presumption in my absense.

"When we were alone together, I would begin to believe what she told me; but, only as long as she gave no sign that she might be in league with another person; which might be as small a thing as speaking to that person; aye, even to look in their direction.

"But she could not fail to draw attention and admiration, wherever she might go, so there were ever connexions of which I was not part, and which must play upon my suspicions. It matter'd not that she refused to reciprocate; the connexion was made, notwithstanding.

"My reason told me that, deny'd all converse, she should have been dull; that, that she might draw no admiration, she must be plain. But my passion contended that she must be bright and beautiful, yet be deny'd converse and admiration.

"'Twas not reasonable, sir, and that plainly so; but, neither was it reasonable that I should enjoy the exclusive affections of such a one as she; so I could not accept them as offer'd, and might have lost her, sir. Aye, more than once, 'twas a close-fought thing."

"But you o'ercame the difficultyes, and stay'd faithful these many years."

"Those difficultyes, aye, and a good many more, sir. 'Tis well that you draw me to speak o't, for 'tis a circumstaunce too little cogitated upon, perhaps.

"She has been my mainstay, sir, There's no denying of that. When the Master was gone, I'd not have continued, without she was by me; I'm sure in that belief. If the despair hadn't done for me, there was plenty others a-waiting on the chance."

His predominance in Johnson's Will cannot but have occasion'd resentments and ill-feeling. "There were those who were not easy about your legacy, I'll warrant."

"Ha! That there were, sir; the Knight, Hawkins, being foremost among them.

"Doctor Johnson was ever a man for a title, which some times could cloud his vision, so that he think a man worthy on that ground alone; as, in my belief, he did in the case of Sir John.

"He must have possess'd some merit, for that His Majesty had thought fit to honour him, but 'twas never discernible to me, sir; and he said such calumnious things about the Doctor, Elizabeth and myself, that Mister Boswell came to question of him too.

"But, as I say, whether owing to his title, or some other thing, the Doctor made him one of the executors of his Will; which he didn't like the essence of, particularly as it related to me; so he tryd to make off with some of the heritaunce. Indeed, there were certain items that he did get away with, so that I was in no doubt of his malice toward myself, and to my late Master's wishes; and was, by no means, up to the task of maintaining my person against such a powerful adversary, even had I not been in the very depths of grief and disarray.

"'Twas then that my Elizabeth show'd her true colours, plain enough for even a blockhead such as I had been to see.

"I should probably have just cower'd in the ante-room at Bolt-Court, until the Bailiff carry me off. But, she was steadfast, and took me in hand, so that we might work, upon the first clear occasion, truly as man and wyfe, in our own exclusive interest, a-serving of no other, as it were to be thenceforward.

"First she puts forward her uncle as undertaker of the funeral business, which, my being the Doctor's chosen beneficiary, the Knight could no-wise gainsay, and was the first opening where our wishes might be known and acted upon; no mean victory, sir, in the face of the number and standing of the opposition rang'd agin us."

"No, indeed, Master Francis. I have encounter'd your Knight, and know him to be a man well suited to the law; an haughty bearing, mix'd with a great capacity for compelling oratory, and an absolute want of flexibility, is my abiding image of him."

"It did much to mollify the grief we all felt, I might tell you. Not only did we feel that we had bested the Knight, but 'twas a unique, and not commercially injurious, opportunity for Elizabeth's uncle to undertake a burial at Westminster Abbey, which put him in such good spirits, we could not but feel for him.

"Elizabeth was not able to attend the funeral, for as well as these other afflictions, one of our children was badly at that time. He died before we mov'd here."

"I'm sorry."

"Nay, sir. 'Tis the Lord's Will. He hath granted us three of our four. We are thankful for that. Mrs. Thrale was granted but four from eleven.

"I give thanks, above all, that Elizabeth has remain'd strong through it. Though she were not with me, I was able to make a good enough show at the service, and to do my dear Doctor Sam credit, only because she was mine.

"And, after that, though there were those who took our part (some, indeed, of the Doctor's closer friends, had been ask'd by him to look out for us, such as Mister Windham), there were more than enough of those with another intention, so that we were besieg'd by people of all sorts, and I was at a loss. Doctor Sam had put in my mind the idea of removing to Lichfield, which I had resolv'd to do, whatever might be consequent to't; but naught in that way could be put in hand until the affairs were settled, before which time I thought I should run mad with the rattling of minor acquaintaunces, trades-people and, begging your pardon, journalists (mainly from the news-papers), vying for our attention.

"Once again, it fell to Elizabeth to impose order upon the situation, which, once again, she did not fail to do; locating, with the assistaunce of her family, an house, far remov'd from the centre of the stage, as the saying is. Such business as the renting of houses no-wise fell within my purview, or sphere of education, as you might imagine, sir. The idea, then, not to speak of the doing of it, would never have enter'd my mind. But Elizabeth had a wider view. She was fitted to adapt to her new station, as I was not; and, if I am, even now, but ill-fitted to't, 'twas a lost cause entirely in mine hands alone!

"She it was then, who initiated our remouval to Smithfield; and she who engag'd another member of her family to act footman and 'repel borders', as we ex-Navy men have it.

"Though 'twere admixt with concern, and grief at last for the child, we had our own home, and none could worry us there. We were especially taken up with the chance that the house was in St. John's street, for I knew that there was such a street here, having visited the Friary with the Doctor, and it seem'd that, even if we were a year or more from coming here, we had made the first step. If it would be long ere we arriv'd, we had, at least, set off.

"We liv'd at that house for nearly two years, and were mostly happy there. It was the scene of our first coming to be a family in our own way. Our son was born the first year, and we call'd him Sam, as there could be no other name."

"Was the child that dy'd your first?"

"No, sir. She still lives, though she is far from strong. Poor Beth was born but a few weeks before Doctor Levet past away, so was already quite a little miss at Smithfield. She was walking and talking ere the Doctor gave leave for Elizabeth and she to join us at Bolt-Court, shortly after the birth of our second child;

which was after he'd had his paralytick stroke, and Mrs. Williams had dyed also."

"That must have been a bad time for your Master, and for yourself."

"It was the beginning of the end, sir, though he was to rally once more. He went through so much at that time that he might have been better not to hang on.

"But he bore every thing with such fortitude as must be an example to us.

"It was high summer, a year before his death, and he had been sitting for his portrait in the day-time (a thing calculated to give a man an excitation, in my view); after which, he had walk'd, without ill-effect, from St. Martins back to Bolt-Court."

"The house-hold had remouv'd then from Johnson's Court," I confirm'd.

"Aye, sir; more than half a dozen years since, soon after the Master return'd from France with Mister and Mrs. Thrale."

"Ah. You have yet to enlighten me with regard to his association with that lady."

"So I have, sir; and enlighten you I will, but I would not instance weakness on his part, before it can be set against his strength. I believe you must understand the full measure of his afflictions, and his stoicism in the face of them, ere you can judge of his capitulations."

"Fairly said, Master Francis. Forgive my interruptions, I prithee."

"Nay, sir; I'm ever a man for the whole story.

"As I say, apart from the sitting for his picture, and the walk back, it was not a day in which he exerted himself much. It was his normal practise to go abroad by night, often walking great distances, and eating much in taverns; but, on that day, he kept to his room in the after-noon, working out varyous plans. He supp'd at home also, upon some flounder I had fresh collected from Billingsgate; which Mrs. De Mullin poach'd according to her own receipt. I remember that, especially, since it was rare for him to have a good word for her, but he was full of praise that night; she joining him at table, as the mistress of the house."

"You did not dine with them."

"My dining, and supping, and all else, was accomplish'd in the servants' quarters, sir. We might all assemble in the parleur, as aforemention'd, when summon'd thither. Other-wise, I kept me to the kitchen, or to an ante-room which was convenient for the answering of the street-door.

"No, sir. I did not dine in company, lest it be company of mine own inviting.

"On that night, the Master dismiss'd me, as soon as the food was layd, having given me leave to go to Elizabeth, and return on the morrow; which was often liberally granted by him, while we were oblig'd to live apart from one another.

"He saw to his own un-dressing; which he did if I were there or not; and put himself to bed ere the chandel brent down.

"He had long experienc'd difficulty in sleeping, occasionally resorting to concoctions from Mister Holder (his apothecary); but, he preferr'd not to increase the measures of these potions, and had lately left them off, lest he become dependent. Mister Holder tryd to persuade him in favour of their continuaunce, but he could not be mov'd upon't; so had return'd to his natural way of sleeping for about two hours and coming wide-awake.

"This time, when he awoke, he felt woolly and un-clear in his head, which put him into a panick, because of his fear of the mad-ness, which was ever with him; and he fell at once to praying to the All-mighty that, what-ever He might visit upon the Doctor's body, He would spare his reason.

"Ever the experimentalist, he put his mind to the composition of some Latin verses of supplication; which he later said were not at all to his usual standard, but that he was aware of their short-comings at the time, which pleas'd him withal, for it shew'd that he had retain'd his critickal facultyes!

"He was then depriv'd of the ability to improuve upon them by the paralytick stroke, which remouv'd from him the power of speech.

"I have thought so long, and regretted so much, with reference to that night; yet, still there remains the guilt that I was not at hand to help him through such an ordeal. He was not a man as was easy in his own company in the normal course; but to be alone when he was at the mercy of the thing he fear'd most must have drawn him nigh to the limit of his enduraunce, with none to call upon.

"Faithfull Servant, sir? Not much in that, I fear.

"Mercifully, though his speech was lost, he was not, in any other way, impair'd, so could apply himself, in his particular way, to his own treatment.

"Presumably acting upon the principle that wine loosens tongues, he set about the imbibing of a quantity of that commodity; which was an happy notion but, I regret to report, lack'd efficacy. What it did succeed in doing for him though, he having not drunk such stuff for a goodly period, was enable him to sleep; which was, perhaps, the best thing possible.

"He awoke with the dawn and once more set himself to reasoning-out his situation, and what might be done about it.

"Enter, some time later, the faithful servant, right pleas'd with himself, as he ever was, fresh from the side of his beloved Elizabeth. Into the room he bursts, noticing nothing amiss. 'The top of the morning, Doctor Sam,' says he. 'Elizabeth and her family send their felicitations, and Becky has learnt to say your name: 'Docker John-John,' which was sure to give him a laugh; instead of which he just stared, in a most beseeching fashion, sir, and claw'd at the air with his hand, which had a crayon in it."

Master Barber's already broken voice became more so at this, and there was a wetness in his black eyes as he continued: "Not at all un-used to his gyrations, I pay'd him no great mind at first; continuing to rattle on about Elizabeth and the child, and how we hoped soon to be able to find somewhere where we might be closer to each other; of which there was no realistick chance, if the Master would not consent to her admission into Bolt-Court.

"I know not how long it took me to come to the realisation that something was troubling him, out of the ordinary, as you might say; but, at length I saw that he was a-holding up of a card with some writing upon it; so I took it from him, and the truth dawn'd.

"All I could do was to panick; which was not much help to him, and would likely be what I should have done had I been there over-night. I cannot tell. But he took my hand to steady it, and directed me to watch what he was now writing, which was a letter to Mister Allen, the printer, that I could deliver to him; for he was a responsible person, who would be capable of making whatever arrangements and organisings might be required.

"His letter shew'd him to be clear in his thoughts and the substaunce of his message, but he had a difficulty about getting the letters in the right order, which frustrated him and made the letter a long time in the writing.

"As was ever the case with him, his fear that his mind was disordered was allay'd by his experimentalist's interest in the phenomenon; so he was able to finish the letter, which I was fearsomely agitated and impatient of, for its delivery was an office for which I was properly fitted, and I could think of naught else to do."

"Were there no doctors involv'd in his care then?"

"Doctor Pepys was the main one at that time, if I remember, sir; though the Master did not all-ways see eye-to-eye with him, being a great one for bleeding in all eventualityes, where the medical man was more for specifick remedyes, and contended that the Master was a-causing of some of his ailments by an excess of bleeding.

"The Master was never really happy with a medical man after poor Doctor Levet was gone. He believ'd, as we all did in the house-hold, that he was worth all the other physickers and chirurgeons to be found in London.

"He's bury'd in St. Bride's church-yard, you know, sir."

"He must have been a worthy man; and most convenient, being lodg'd on the premises all those years. I well remember reading an account of him published in that Magazine to which I am contributor. 'Twas much to be regretted that he was not still among you at the time of Doctor Johnson's extremity, for he would surely have been equipt to be of service; in which regard, you must cease to chastise yourself, Master Francis, for, as you have owned, it is likely that you could have done little to ameliorate affairs."

"'Tis another case where reason and passion are at odds, sir. My reason would have deserted me, I've little doubt, but my heart would wish to be with him, notwithstanding."

"I understand you; and, though you treat yourself hard, with your sarcastick talk of the faithful servant, none can doubt your love and concern for your late Master. 'Tis that fact that is recognised in the epithet, to be sure. You have reason to be proud of it, friend, and should not turn it against yourself." This was a genuine sentiment which I felt un-able to suppress, and was glad to see the raising of spirits that it brought about in my worthy guest.

"How long did your Master remain thus afflicted? Were the practitioners able to assist him?"

"He-wanted but little assistaunce, sir, for he soon restor'd himself; though he had been much weaken'd by the affair, and was un-able to speak for long periods together, without his voice deserted of him a-fresh.

"But, within a week, he was up to attending church, and dining with the Club. He even, in despite of all the years he had spent a-convincing of us that it made no difference, went and took the aire at Hampstead, follow'd by two weeks away at Mister Langton's house at Rochester, for the same purpose. His friends were very good and solicitous about him, especially Mrs. Davies, the book-seller's wyfe, who was a good woman, and an excellent friend to all who knew her.

"While he was at Rochester, he made several outings to see such as the Chatham Docks; and soon after went to stay with Mister Bowles in Salisbury Heale; there being no mor'n about six weeks from the stroke to the full restoration of his constitution."

"Marvellous! What a man!"

"Aye, sir; a man, indeed; but one whose afflictions were only just beginning."

CHAPTER TWELVE

IN WHICH THE DOCTOR IS FURTHER AFFLICTED AND WE HEAR ABOUT SOME CELEBRATED CALLERS AT BOLT COURT

"A close bond had form'd between the Doctor and Mrs. Williams in the time that they had liv'd under the same roof. She was a woman of wide interests and knowledge who was capable of conversing on a level with him. Also, unlike myself, she was not afraid to voice her opinions in his presence.

"I ever found her peevish and ill-dispos'd, but they spent many hours in company, dining, supping, talking and laughing.

"While she was still capable o't, he would even take her abroad with him, when he went a-visiting, in and around Fleet Street; which could be something of a spectacle, sir, The Doctor, as previously describ'd could be sufficient of same, un-accompanyed; but the addition of an ancient blind woman to the scene had people quite falling down with mirth.

"When Doctor Sam took it upon himself to have one of his gyrations in the street, Williams would be let loose, so that she grop'd about, a-pawing of the air, trying to re-establish a grip upon him; but until the gyrations ran their course, there were no part of him as would stay still long enough that she should retain her hold. By that time, the urchins would join in, some a groping; others gyrating, and all-together making the most merrye goings-on.

"People as they visited were never depriv'd of this entertainment, for Doctor Sam had an invariable gyration he perform'd when entering an house. It had some connexion with his business of counting the tethering posts, and I think may have proceeded from a long held superstition. What-ever 'twas, it requir'd him all ways to enter upon the right foot; along with which, he must thrash the air with. his arms and, more often than not, revolve upon his axis, as it were. I have a sort of memory of something like it in my Jamaican life, but 'twas un-Christian; some matter of 'evil spirits'; I know not.

"As in the street, when the gyration commenced, poor Jenny

would be cast adrift; and it was chance alone, on more than one occasion, as prevented her falling downstair.

"Like the Doctor, she had a sort of pre-visitation of the malady that carry'd her off, five or six years earlier, from which she seem'd to mend; but, by the time of the Master's stroke, she was in her chamber at Bolt-Court, in a pathetick way, e'en her temper still'd.

"Doctor Brocklesby was in attendaunce, a-confining of his skills for the most to alleviation, having no great hopes of recovery; in fact, he had no expectation that she would again quit her chamber alive. For all that that was the diagnosis, he said her decay was likely to be a slow, drawn out process, and she seem'd to be still with us in mind, so that her demise should not be imminent.

"I was little about her in those days. Betsy (that's Mrs. White, the maid-servant) look'd after her wants; and there was Poll to call upon in need ."

"Poll?"

"Carmichael; Poll Carmichael, sir. The Doctor took her in out of charitye, I believe, for she was but little use about the place. She was just deliver'd to us by him one day, along with the information that she would be a-joining of us. De Mullin fair exploded upon receipt thereof, saying, quite rightly, that there was more than enough people employ'd about the business of the house as it was, especially had any on them been much good for any thing." He put on an high-pitch'd and affected voice:

"'And where, pray, is the creature to sleep?' says she, regarding poor Poll as if she had been a cock-roach. 'Hi 'ave some pride left, heven hif hi *ham* a poor widow, whose dear 'usband as gorn orn afore. Hi'll not share my bed with the likes of she, and there's a hend hon't!'

"Then Poll starts: 'Ah've nae desyre tae sleep wi' ye, neither, ye stupet au'd wimman! Prade, ess et? Well, see me; ah've go' ma prade 'n' a',' and she goes for De Mullin's throte, sir.

"Betsy and I are both standing by, bethinking 'tis the jollyest sport imaginable; but the Master calms 'em down, holding Poll off De Mullin, which last looks like she's up for the vapours, and bringing them to sit down, the table betwixt them, while a solution is arriv'd at.

"At length, all things having been consider'd, there's but one course to be taken. There was, up to then, a sort of guest-chamber, which Mister Boswell was used to have at his disposition. With the increase in the in-mates, this was to become the female-servants' dormitory; to which end, *some one* must be put to the carrying of the beds and movables, sir."

"So Poll and Betsy mov'd up into the house proper?"

"Aye, and De Mullin too, sir.

"So it was that these three women were to be found together in that room; they all being better fitted to wait upon Mrs. Williams than myself.

"I should say, as an aside, sir, that Mister Boswell receiv'd of the idea that De Mullin had a daughter that was one of the incumbents of the dormitory, and recorded such a notion in his *Life*. He was mis-taken in this; there being no daughter, though she did have a son: John, who was a good young man, and helpt me much in the last days of the Doctor, as you shall hear; Doctor Johnson leaving him an annuitye in his Will.

"The only people in that room, other than De Mullin, were Betsy and Poll; and, daughter or no, De Mullin had flounc'd off after a falling out with Mrs. Williams, so was not there neither.

"Be that as it may, sir; how it was to come out was a surprise to us all, Doctor Brocklesby included; but Mrs. Williams declin'd to take her food soon after the Doctor left for Wiltshire.

"She had ever a singular diet; the greater part of which consisted of bread and butter; and her main delicacyes being oysters and porter, to which she attributed her long life. And long 'twere, sir, but she could not claim much benefit to health for it.

"The long and the short of it was that she dyed while the Doctor was yet at Salisbury; which was blow upon blow for him, as you might say.

"He had no such feeling for any of the others in the house as he had for that woman, and for Doctor Levet; and they were both now gone from him, so that he felt bereft of friends."

"But you were still there, were you not?"

"Of course, sir; and I was busyer about him than I had ever been; but I was also marryd, so that Elizabeth must occupy as much of my time and thoughts as could be spared. Accordingly, whilst he was away, sir, so was I. When he return'd, which was soon after Mrs. Williams's passing, he was extremely ill-humour'd, so I kept out of his way."

"Did his sense of loss bring back the hypochondria?"

"In sooth, sir, it did not; for he was too angry to become melancholick. Though he had recover'd from the stroke, still he was plagu'd with the gout; and he had acquir'd a new affliction, which was not to be spoken of, but which gave him great inconvenience, and would have need of the chirurgeon's knife for its removal."

"What was it then?" I ask'd.

He pull'd a frightful face before replying: "A *sarockle*, sir."

"A what?"

"A sarockle. It's a lump, sir; as it would be a tumour, on a man's *particular parts*, if you follow me."

"Ah. A *sarco-cele*, a tumour of the muscle-tissues."

"What-ever it be call'd, I'd as lief move on to another topick, as summarily as may be, sir. The Master bore the thing with great fortitude, and was prepared, in every way, for the necessarily tormentous business of its amputation; but the doctors were in no such haste, and fell instead to muttering together in a learned and scientifick way, such that, 'twas my belief they would have kept him and his *sarockle* for an exhibition."

"It is to be imagined that they fear'd for the effects upon Johnson of the operation, so put it off as long as they were able."

"You may be right in that, sir; but *I* form'd the idea that their medical sensibilityes were excited by it, and that they would watch it for as long as they could, to see what it would do next; in which it frustrated and dis-appointed them, sir, by vanishing of its own volition!

"Soon after this, we receiv'd a special guest at Bolt-Court, I answering the door to her. Who do you think, sir? You'll never be able to guess, I'll wager. None other than Mrs. Siddons, sir, the toast of the London stage; but as un-affected a woman as you might meet.

"The Master was still sore afflicted with the gout, so it fell to me to conduct her to her carriage, where, handing her in, I found that she had taken notice of me: 'Bless you, Frank,' says she. 'Mind you take good care of your Master; and, perhaps he will take you one day to see me in the theatre'; whereupon she gave me a shilling, sir."

"What? A shilling? Vulgar show!"

"Not at all, sir. There was none of-the vulgar about her, which surpriz'd the Master, he being no lover of actors in the normal way.

"No, sir; she behaved in every way as a lady should; and, if her success was such as she could part with a shilling to the likes of me, 'twas a token well meant; and well receiv'd too, sir."

"Were there any other callers to the house that impress'd you?"

"There were many, sir, to be sure; though few on the grounds of fame or blood. The Doctor being a good man, he seem'd to draw others of that kind about him, albeit they often came through some connexion with printing or literature.

"One such was Mrs. Gardiner, who dyed about three years since. She was the wyfe of a tallow-chandler on Snow-Hill, not in the learned way, but a worthy good woman, and a regular caller from the early days, having been introduced to the Doctor by Mrs. Masters, the poetess."

"Mary Masters."

"That is she, sir; and Mrs. Ann Gardiner. 'Twas after her we named our youngest. She establish'd a school for the poor, as I might; though hers was singular in being restricted to the education of females, about which she had rather advanc'd ideas.

"If I can't write like the Doctor, and I can't heal the sick like Mister Levet, I might, at least, found a school, like Mrs. Gardiner, sir. What think you?"

"I think the purpose does you credit; and I'm sure you will do honour to all of them."

"I thank you for the sentiment, sir. I shall certainly do my best in that regard."

"No more could be ask'd of any man."

He look'd at me in his penetrating way for a moment or two; then made a bow with his head, before returning to the contemplation of the scene. The promenade would soon be upon us, and the sun was getting low, the cool zephyrs of dusk bringing thoughts of another move.

"Another caller of whom I was fond was Miss Burney, for all that she all-ways addrest me as *Blacky*; something I should not welcome from most people.

"I read her *Evelina* when it first came out. She was not so shallow as many of the others. She had a writer's mind, so that she could see things below the surface, and understand other ways of looking than her own.

"She was very kind to me, sir; was all-ways afraid to put me to too much trouble. Though, 'tis certainly true that she could be infuriating – often from that very refusal to put a man to trouble which he does not deem to be trouble, so that it were more trouble to ascertain what she would have done, than would be the-doing of it!"

"I think I follow you, Master Francis."

"And she could also be silly, in that way which was (more then than now) seen as witty and amusing; at which times there was no sense to be got from her. 'Twas like old Mister Foote, the comedian, who would oft say a thing because it was laughable, or ridiculous, rather than in the strict interests of veracity.

"Doctor Sam, for all he claim'd other-wise, was not entirely free of this practise; being more driven by the turning of a pritty phrase than would be strictly in the cause of accuracy. Miss Burney had not his immediacy of sensibility, so could be carry'd away by her own wit to a degree that would quite make a man despair, sir."

CHAPTER THIRTEEN

IN WHICH MASTER BARBER TALKS OF MOVING ON; RELATES
THE TALE OF SHAKESPEARE'S MULBERRY TREE, AND PRESENTS
US TO A MOST SINGULAR PERSONAGE

"I'm beginning to feel the chill, Master Francis, and have no desire to fall in with the promenade, our private converse pleasing me much. What think you of repairing to some fire-lit interior?"

"I am in your hands, and at your service, Master Reporter; but I cannot deny that my throte is in want of lubrification."

"Well, then, let us find a fire and some refreshment." I sprang up and assisted Master Barber to his feet.

The first of the townes-people had reach'd our end of the Pool, so it was mete that we should be off. Facing us, at the point where the track by St. Chad's joins Stow-street, there is a second stately house; occupying the same eminence as Stow House, but lower down, upon the wester side, so as to be isolated by the rise. "What house is that?" My research being found wanting in its respect, I put the question to my companion.

"It is the *sister-house* to Stow-Hill, sir. The two houses were residences of the two Aston sisters, who shared the Hill, and the adjoining park, but kept their separate houses.

"Miss Aston liv'd in the upper house, and Mrs. Gastrel in the lower; she being the widow of the Reverend Mister Gastrel, who once had the charge of Shakespeare's Garden at Stratford-upon-Avon. Mister Boswell says that they were responsible for the cutting-down of the Bard's mulberry tree in the course of their tenure. I think they were tired by all the criticisms and questions of people who visited the garden. Concluding they could do nothing right, they thought they might as well do something positively *wrong*, so cut down the tree; which I should think would be most effectual in silencing the rattle; albeit for an abbreviated period!"

"Indeed; indeed!"

"Mister Boswell describ'd the affair, from the view-point of the Shakespeare enthousiast, as an instance of sacrilege. The test of that will have been made, now that both the Reverend and Mrs. G. have been call'd to account, sir ."

"So, Mrs. Gastrel is no more?"

"No, sir; though she is much mourn'd, not least by my wyfe and myself, who have been more than a little inconvenienced by her passing."

"Why so?"

"'Twas from her that we rented the house in which we have liv'd since our removal from London; she and her sister having built the houses at this end of Stow-street. With her demise has come a great deal of confusion as to who owns what, and we have been under sufferaunce here for nigh on two years as a result.

"It is a goodly house, and serves us very well, but we are now given notice, so will likely remove to an house amenable to the accommodation of a school, if something can be found to rent. The rents are more manageable in the villages and hamlets round about than they are in the citye, so we may be forced to quit St. Chad's all together."

We had made progress along Stow-street as we talk'd, and now came to the house, which was part of a row of such; flat-fronted, but not without character. One side of it o'er-reached a wynd, which gave access to a spinney; from whence the land rose toward St. Michael's Church, where we had passed earlier in the after-noon.

Master Barber bade me forgive his lack of hospitalitye, his kitchen being un-prepared for my arrival here; which I could not hold to be dis-courteous. 'Twas true that he had no notice of my visit, and I had suggested no desyre to impose upon him or his familye. I told him, rather, that I should consider it an honour if Mrs. Barber could sup with us; which had been true if there were time at my disposal, so that we had liberty to pursue nicetyes and light discourse; but my true purpose was best-serv'd by having my guest all-undivided.

He return'd that he consider'd it a most genteel offer, but

that his wyfe could not possibly leave Beth and the other children.

He then begg'd my leave to go into the house and advyse his wyfe of his doings, inviting me to stand in the vestibule; but I declin'd, being minded to respect his and his wyfe's privacy.

Two cats station'd themselves at the street end of the wynd, to regard this stranger curiously, as I attended my companion's re-appearaunce. When I addrest them, one presented itself for stroking, whilst the other snubb'd me and saunter'd off across the street. I stood in a patch of red sunlight, the last blaze of evening, and gazed along the street the way we had lately come. The houses opposite were become silhouettes, and the road-way had already that sheen that comes upon it by night. There was no wheel'd traffick, and very little motion of any sort on that Sabbath eve. A matron was sweeping before her house with a besom; some dogs were scavenging in the courts and wynds, and the spinneys were alive with bird-song. As they had done some hours before, the bells now broke upon the aire; this time summoning the faithful to even-song.

The door of the house open'd at last, creaking loudly as it did so. I advanced to re-unite with my friend and found he was not alone, Mrs Elizabeth Barber having come out to make my acquaintaunce.

Master Francis presented me to her as nicely as you please, and she gave a most decorous curtsey. She was indeed a handsome woman (something around the forty of years, I should guess), though perhaps a little thin and peaky. Akin to her husband in stature, though very straight to his tendency to stoop, she shared his scrubb'd cleanliness, but far o'er-reach'd him in dress. It may be that she hastily donn'd this raiment on being appris'd of my presence, though she look'd not to have been created in haste.

If 'twere not so, she is one for dressing right prittily for the doing of house-work. Both her cap and her gown were money, Dear Reader; naught here of the cast-off; this stuff was of the finest, and *for* the finest.

"I am most grate-full to you, sir, for the interest you take in my husband. I'm sure that you will employ your highest judgement and discretion in recording what passes between you.

"Our lives have seen us high and low by turns, and we expect no alteration to the pattern hereafter. Our connexions to the wise have given us enough of wisdom to fulfil our destiny, and to pass on such as we have to others.

"If some record of our being goes forward, it is all that we can ask.

"If any should learn from such record that our love was possible, and enduring, and honourable; that our errours have been from simplicitye, rather than sin; that men and women need not dye as they are born, but may try other lands, or other lives, where travail and compensation are in better balance; if any should come to learn that the real oppressor is ignorance, sir (for, without it, the fancy'd oppressor is un-arm'd); If any of these things should come of it, I say, then it is a thing well done.

"Your servant, sir. God be with you."

She curtsey'd again, kiss'd Master Francis, and was gone, the heavy door thudding behind her. Her voice, and the intensitye with which she had deliver'd of these sentiments had held me as in a spell, and I had utter'd no word to her throughout.

The vision of her has remain'd with me, standing upon the step in the red blaze of the sun, like an angel speaking down the ages. There was about her an inner strength and determination, which came from, and went on beyond, her present existence (or so I deem'd it), as if she had liv'd this life as proof of some principle which might be adopted in another, and by others, with more reward. She made an impression upon me, you may be sure, as few others have ever done; though I have been no stranger to the *great* and the *good*. In short, I perceiv'd in her *nobility* of a quality and a measure not to be found in most who are held to satisfye the imperatives of the term.

I had much to think upon as Master Francis once more fell in with me, and we set off, in silence, in the direction of the High Cross.

CHAPTER FOURTEEN

IN WHICH MASTER BARBER WEIGHS HIS BLESSINGS AND
TRIBULATIONS, REPORTS SOME IMPROPRIETIES BY A KNIGHT
OF THE REALM, AND ACCOMPANIES HIS MASTER ON A 'JAUNT'
TO OXFORD

Though Lichfield boasts many fine inns and tavernes, and
though 'twould be a great pleasure to sample 'em all,
'twere both more politick and more prudent to return to the
Swan for our evening repast; my status as a resident ensuring a
table, and the eventualitye of there being but a single reckoning
for bed and board facilitating negociation.

Master Barber remain'd silent and pensive until we reach'd
the cross. As we left Stow-street, and came into Tamworth-
street, he seem'd to return to himself.

"You have met my wyfe, then, sir."

I must needs say something to this, expressive of my
(genuine and profound) admiration, but un-provoking to my
friend's jalousye. "She hath a rare beautye, and exquisite
bearing, Master Francis; possessing at the same time fine
sensibilityes and intellect. I confess myself most affected by our
meeting. She must be a great blessing and a consolation to you
in your tribulations."

"A blessing she is, indeed, sir; and that of greater magnitude
than a man such as I could dare to hope for.

"My early life has led me to the contemplation of things in a
nautical light, sir; a sort of method for determining your
bearings, as it were. View'd that way, Elizabeth is my anchor,
my haven, my wind, my sea, my sun, my stars, aye, and my very
vessel. In short, she is my life.

"A blessing, sir? That she is, aye, and a consolation too.

"But, sir, a man can find strength enough to support his
tribulations, for he hath no other course.

"Where is he to find reserves enough to support such a
consolation?"

I did not reply to this curious question, for I had no answer and, in any event, 'twas not expected; but I reflected that a surfeit of gifts may not be without a concomitant share of liabilityes.

We resum'd our silence now, as we continued past the fountain into Bore-street, speaking only in reply to such citizens as bade us "Good-evening," most of whom addrest Master Francis by name.

In Bore-street, a vendor was selling roasted chestnuts from a brazier, the aroma of which hung upon the evening aire in a most appetizing way, while the flickering gave an element of excitement and up-lift to the scene. I had almost resolv'd to begin treating with the vendor, when I recall'd the indentate condition of my companion, and abandon'd the notion.

In the street, knots of townes-folk gather'd to converse. In a charming; rustick way, the habitaunts of a row, or court, congregate in the street, then move off, all in a body, to church, the Minster, or a place of entertainment.

We soon came out by the Friary and, turning right, were back upon Bird-street. Before we enter'd the Swan, my companion arrested me. "Forgive me if I have been something sullen and un-companionable since Stow-street, sir.

"When I tell you of my life, it raises my spirits considerably; but, when I look upon my child, it ever brings me up short."

"I understand, friend. How does Mistress Beth?"

"She bears up bravely, sir. She has days when she is much better, but it seems she must ever pay for them with days such as she now has."

"What do the doctors think it is?"

"A *judgement*, sir."

"I intended that you should understand *medical* doctors, by my question."

"So I did, sir. They talk of other things, and they prescribe concoctions of every sort for her treatment, leading to ruinous trade with the apothecaryes; but ask what they think it is, and I have answer'd you truthfully.

"Still, sir; it was not for this that I stopt you ere we went with-in.

"I am your guest; and right hospitably treated as such; so that it does not behove me to dwell upon such quotidian matters. I am aware of my duty as guest to supply good and entertaining companye, and it is to apprise you of which that I hold you here.

"Once we enter the inn, I shall dwell no longer upon the present, and return happily to the past."

"Be assured that I am sensible of the matter that exercises you at this time. If you utter'd not another word to me, I should have been amply repaid for a dinner and a supper. I thank you heartily for your time; and I would have your wyfe thank'd for allowing it.

"Come ye in, Master Francis, and be ye merry, for that it can make no situation the worse, and may re-invigourate ye much." I patted his shoulder companionably, and we went in.

The interior was somewhat rowdyer than we had left it earlier in the day; the cause of which being the return of the mechanicks and labourers currently engag'd upon alterations to the Swan. Having suspended operations for the Sabbath, they must re-commence on the morrow, so, having come back from visits to their familyes, or varyous carousings closer-by, they now seem'd intent upon making themselves sufficiently insensible to sleep in the stables.

The table we had occupy'd at dinner was free, however, and was well-remov'd from the clamour of the publick rooms, so we resum'd our positions there, and I call'd for some claret.

"The house-hold must have been very different, with Mister Levet, Mrs. Williams and Mrs. Desmoulins *all* gone," I suggested, when once we were properly install'd.

"We were return'd to the position that we occupy'd at Inner Temple Lane, sir, but for Betsy and Poll, of course. The strange outcome was that I became senior-man, as it were, where the domestick arrangements were concern'd. Whereas theretofore I had been accus'd of all that was amiss, I was become 'clerk of the kitchen'!

"But that was as nothing to me, compared to my moving back to first rank with my Master. When Williams had been there, and De Mullin, they had been his *confidantes,* and his general society. Back in the days at Inner Temple, I had perform'd that function; being then more like a son than at any other time.

"Now, not only did he consent to Elizabeth and the children joining me, but he began again to take an interest in me, as if I had slipp'd from his mind in the intervening years, and he, of a sudden, remember'd who I was.

"He reviv'd his interest in my education, too. He was well pleas'd with my command of language and my general standard, but sayd that I was wanting in *breadth* of knowledge, having spent too much of my reading upon works of romance and fiction.

"He decided to rectify this situation, by giving me a course of reading of an encyclopædic nature; so I was despatched with a letter to Mister Dilly's book-shop in the Poultry, with a view to procuring a set of *Burton's Books.* Doctor Sam remembered having seen them in the old book-shop on London Bridge, and thought there were about five or six in a set, instead of which there were more than thirty! But they dealt with such a wide sweep of topicks, that they greatly expanded my *general* knowledge, in a manner that application to each topick in turn would take a life-time to achieve.

"I was proud of those books, which were mine, and bought for me by the Doctor. He allocated a section of his book-shelves for them, as they were mine own personal library; and I was very careful of their preservation, for the Doctor was a devourer of books. When he had extracted the meaning and the information from them, he seemed to have gone to their very marrow, so that they were hollowe and broken. I wanted my books to hold their perfection ."

"Do you keep them still to pass to your children?"

His voice and his manner betray'd something like anger, or bitter-ness, in responding to this question. "No, sir. I do not.

"In his Will, Doctor Johnson gave certain of his books to those he thought would benefit from them. He also allow'd such as Mrs. Gardiner to choose what they would from his library, so that they might each have a volume to remember him by.

"He did not, however, make any specifick direction with regard to the rest of the library, on the understanding that it should all come to me.

"The Knight, in his wisdom, determin'd that I should have no use for reading or learning, and succeeded in persuading Sir Joshua and Doctor Scott likewise, so that I think he took what he would have for himself, and the rest was sold by auction; but that I had no ground for complaint under the law (or otherwise), because the proceeds of the sale went into the fund."

"But this was o'er-stepping their authority as executors; that they should act where there was no specifick instruction."

"That is so, sir; but the Knight had not the cerebration to be dis-interested.

"He could not execute the wishes of the Master unless they should conform to his wishes. When he deem'd them contrary to his own method of thinking, yet was still oblig'd to carry them out, he would pay himself a forfeit, so that, by no matter how little, he had altered the Will of the Master in that matter.

"And, it was essentially as it should benefit me that he discern'd contrariety in't."

"You were surely wrong'd, Master Francis; and I wonder, for all that, that none stood your corner on these matters. Was it not Johnson's purpose in detailing certain of his friends to your protection?"

"I'm sure it was, sir; but, it must be comprehended that *protection* may take as many forms as there are partyes interested in it.

"When you have charge of a small child, or an ideot, you will oft deem it prudent to protect it from its self. Convinced of your own superiority of experience and intellect, you will make its decisions for it; the authority of age and size carrying the argument on every occasion.

"Although I was a man of forty years, of which more than thirty had been spent with the Doctor; and, though he had exprest his wishes direct to me, the primary of which being that I continue to expand my knowledge; still those who come from outside must apply their prejudice to the affair.

"Only Sir John's romantick view of English candour allow'd the *general* tenour of the Will to go forward. He, and his shrew of a daughter, had a divine conviction of their superiority that would not submit to any testing, for that they lack'd both the apprehension and the inclination to alter it; so that any action taken against me was justify'd by rules of their own making.

"An animal sees no further than its own interest. A man might be expected to have somewhat more of vision.

"A man is a man, whether he be born a slave or a King; and, for all that you dress it up in fine cloaths and call it 'sir', an animal rests an animal.

"I know not if it still persists, but there was a theory abroad some years since that the *orang-outan* is a man, because it *looks* like one. We need not wonder long at the advancement of Sir J. H. with that in mind, methinks."

"Ho, sir! Cru-ell, cru-ell! But not un-call'd for; not at all!"

"The others that were charg'd with our looking-after by the Doctor were persuaded that our best interests were being serv'd; because they, similarly, form'd their own ideas of what those best interests would be, without application to our judgement.

"They also had firm ideas as to the *outcome* of bequeathing such a legacy to the likes of us, so were ever industrious in its coming to pass; for it's a much easier course to fit the world to your notions, than to fit your notions to the world. Is that not so, Master Reporter?"

"Hah ! And what would you expect a journalist to say to that, sir? The very idea!" This succeeded in allaying his anger, for he saw its ironick intent at once; a broad smile comeing to his gummy mouth. I was doubley pleas'd at this for, though he intended other-wise, he had not, until then, shaken off the mood of melancholy that had descended when we visited his house in Stow-street.

I replenysh'd our goblets, and he took up the account of Johnson's last year at Bolt-Court.

"With the arrival of winter, the Master's afflictions began to gather around him a-new; appearing first as a catarrhal cough, which, in turn precipitated asthma of such virulence that he was not able to lie at night, but must be helpt to sit up. He was also visited with the dropsy, so that it was ever more difficult for him to move, or be mov'd.

"Not long before Christmas it was, that he was confin'd to the house, and look'd not likely to leave.

"It even became necessary to turn away such as Mister Perkins and his wyfe."

"Perkins?"

"He as ran Thrale's Brewery, after the passing of old Mister T., sir. He call'd occasionally with his wyfe and Children, but the Master was too indispos'd to see them at that time.

"Doctor Brocklesby's view was that the return of fine weather would bring relief; which was not an early prospect in London, in January; so the Master took a notion to go to Italy, where he might find a better climate and better aire the sooner; and he communicated this idea to Mister Boswell. That person thought it such an excellent notion that he made plans to come to London and set the matter in hand. He also, at the Master's request, ask'd the advise of some of his physicians as to whether 'twas the right course, or what else might be suggested.

"The Doctor had become so bad at this time that I thought his end was nigh. He was barely recognizable, either in his look, or in his voice. But then, of a sudden, I heard shouts from his chamber, when he had sent me upon an errand.

"Bounding up the stair, I threw open the door to be met with an astonishing scene. The swelling of his legs was no more; he having dis-charg'd full twenty pints of water.

"By the end of February, his asthma had also abated, and he was return'd to taking an interest in the world.

"Varyous packets and letters then began to arrive from the learned medical men that Mister Boswell had consulted; but, by that time, the Master was well on the track to recovery; Doctor Heberden having join'd Doctor Brocklesby in his attention.

"In the event, Mister Boswell did not arrive in London, having turn'd back with a view to entering Parliament, and the

Italy jaunt was not to come off, neither.

"Instead, I was to have much of Doctor Johnson's companye, for he was un-able to go abroad until the end of April, having been five months confin'd.

"During that period we were much together, and he came to know Elizabeth, as he had not before; appreciating her great intelligence and personal qualityes, in addition to her prittiness and presentability, which he had remark'd upon before.

"Indeed, so partial to her did he become, that he invested in her a valuable mementoe of himself, the character of which I cannot divulge to you, for he put her and me upon oath in that regard; but that it is an object of veneration, whose existence remains un-guess'd at by such as the Knight, who bethink themselves so superior; but was given to my wyfe."

I did not wish him to think too much upon the Knight, that he should revert to his previous low spirits, but I could not let this intelligence pass without I made some try at drawing him out upon't.

"Did I not hear somewhere of this? Surely 'twas a ring; as you say, of some value to Johnson, that your wyfe now has."

"Nay, sir; there is such a ring, which I won't deny; but given by myself to Elizabeth. It had previously belonged to Mrs. Johnson, and was kept by the Master as a token of her.

"On his passing, I offer'd it to Miss Porter, her daughter, here in Lichfield, but she wanted nothing of it, being out of sorts at receiving nothing direct from the Doctor's hand, as you might say, he having omitted her from the Will. 'Twas odd that she should take it so amiss, having neglected similarly to leave aught to him, though her Will was made while he yet liv'd. She, too, is gone now, having dyed the following year.

"As to the ring, I took it to be enamell'd. It had been Mrs. Johnson's wedding ring, but I had it made into a mourning ring for the Master, and gave it to Elizabeth."

"A most fitting deed, Master Francis; but that, you say, is not the object to which you earlier alluded."

"It is not, sir; and I would beg you to seek no further after the details thereof, for it is a matter of sacred trust with my

Master, and I have already cause to regret the mention I made of it, which was only to convey the measure of regard in which the Master held my Elizabeth."

"Then we shall speak of it no more, for I respect both your confidence and your faithfulness to your Master; but, since you yourself planted the seeds of curiosity, you must allow that I cannot easily dismiss the matter from my mind."

"I say this to still your curiosity, though I fear it might further inflame it: unless you are already appris'd of the existence of the object under discussion, I'm certain that you shall not be able to guess at it."

I could say no more to that, though I have often in idle moments cogitated upon the possible nature of Johnson's gift. The more time I have dedicated to speculation, the less clear I am about the kind or sort of thing it could have been. I can hardly think that it was very valuable, though Master Francis said it was. What is valuable to one man may be less so to another. What's more, there is monetary value; there is sentimental value, and there is the value placed upon an object by *posterity*. Any thing which belong'd to Doctor Johnson would be possess'd of intrinsick value. There are already collectors avid for items with a proven Johnsonian connexion.

But all of this avail'd me naught. One day, no doubt, the object will come to light, and what must remain a riddle in this journal shall at last be solv'd.

Supper at the Swan was to be jugg'd hare or game pye, and we both settled upon the former, having been inform'd that the hares were local-cours'd upon Dimbles-Hill, a fortnight since, and hung on the premises.

I am pleas'd to relate that my guest's humour did not suffer by my inquisitiveness, or his contemplation, of the Knight. The claret was going down right well, and the thought of the hare seem'd to raise him still further.

I directed that more claret of the same batch be put in readyness, and bade Master Francis continue.

"By the time Mister Boswell came at last to London in May, the Master was almost fully restor'd. We had a succession of visitors and well-wishers, until it became difficult for Elizabeth and myself to cope, with only Poll and Betsy to call on; though, at least the Doctor was now able to go abroad again, so that he was often entertain'd at other houses. As soon as we could, we prevail'd upon De Mullin to re-join the house-hold for, with Williams gone, there was none left to vex her – even myself, for I was much better behav'd in Elizabeth's presence!

"Of course, she had fallings-out with Poll, which we all did; finally resulting in the Scotch wench's turning out; which we were sorry for, for she was no more argumentative and no less use last than first; so that I thought she should have been throw'n out right away, or kept to the end.

"By June, the Doctor was well enough to contemplate travelling, and decided to visit Oxford, in which Mister Boswell (and myself) would accompany him. I reserv'd the places for Mister Boswell and the Master on the stage-coach, the day before departure, arranging to come behind in the heavy-coach with the valises.

"We stay'd at that place a fortnight together, the most of which was spent in. company with Mister Adams and others of the Doctor's long acquaintaunce.

"It was also upon this jaunt, though I knew naught of it, until I should read it in Mister Boswell's *Life*, that my annuity, and the sum of it, were discuss'd – upon the publick stage-coach!"

CHAPTER FIFTEEN

IN WHICH MASTER BARBER DISCOURSES ON THE SUBJECT OF
BIOGRAPHY, AND DELIVERS CERTAIN REVELATIONS IN THE
MATTER OF HIS MASTER AND MRS. THRALE

"It was wonderful to see how well the Master supported himself in Oxford, having been all that time confin'd to Bolt-Court. He held his ground in debate as ever; his mind still fresh and growing, for all that he had suffer'd in body.

"Even on the journey there, he had given good value. I had book'd the seats in his and Mister Boswell's names, as the Doctor bethought himself liable to queasyness from counter-movement, so desir'd that the for'ard facing seats be specifically reserv'd.

"Accordingly, their fellow-travellers could identifye them from the way-bill; they being an American woman and her daughter, if I recall aright. One of them, being American, ask'd outright if the Master was 'the *famous* Doctor Johnson', as soon as he boarded the coach. Knowing who he was, so not without expectation, still she marvell'd at his talk, saying that 'every sentence was an essay'.

"Many subjects were treated of in the course of this jaunt, from Milton to Pope, the rich to the poor, and back again, sir. We saw much of Oxford, which is a magnificent place, sir, if you have not been that way."

"So I believe,"I told him, tho' 'twas far from un-familiar to me.

"It was suggested that the Doctor produce a prayer-book, which he had neither time, nor *vitalitye* to consider, but he was pleas'd that it should be put forward.

"All-in-all, for as long as we rested there, he kept himself up to the mark. But, once in the coach for the return to London, the demand to give out being gone, he became very tired, and seem'd not very well."

"The man must have been exhausted."

"I'm sure he was, sir; but he shew'd no improuvement in the

following weeks; nor much inclination to rest. A week later, he was present at the Literary Club; about him, Mister Boswell, Lord *This* and Bishop *That* – men of great moment of whom I can recall naught.

"The deterioration in him was generally recogniz'd there and elsewhere, by his friends and companye, so that they heartily endors'd the idea of a jaunt to Italy, which indeed the Master had come ever more enthousiastick about, knowing, as we all did in our hearts, that he should not survive a further winter at Bolt-Court.

"Unbeknownst to us all, Mister Boswell had prosecuted a plan on behalf of those friends of his to secure the money necessary for the undertaking from the Lord Chancellor. Obtaining a favourable initial response from that quarter, he arriv'd in some excitation at Bolt-Court, where he found the Doctor somewhat improuv'd. 'I'm very anxious about you, sir, and particularly that you should go to Italy for the winter, which I believe is your own wish,' says Boswell. 'You have no objection, I presume, but the money it would require.' He then shew'd him the letter from Mister Edward Thurlow, the Lord Chancellor, and told him what had gone forward on his behalf.

"The Master was so mov'd by this that he could not contain his agitation, and began to cry. 'This is taking prodigious pains about a man,' says he. 'God bless you all.' At which, Mister Boswell is similarly reduced to lachrymation; and I don't know whether to laugh, or join them."

"Laugh? Why so?"

"Relief, sir; or, perhaps, glee. I know not; for, in truth, I know not if I was happy about the idea of his going.

"I need not tell you that I wish'd him the best thing possible. If Italy would afford him relief or longevity, I was all for it. But I did not wish to be parted from him, having restor'd fully the mutuality of our affection and respect; particularly should it be for the last time, as I could not but fear that it should be.

"If sufficient were found that I should, accompany him, 'twas well and good; and right that I, of all people, should be at his side there. Such wonders, I believe there are in Italy, that we would do very well, in conformity with the pattern we had lately re-establish'd.

"For all that there were in its favour, there was now my Elizabeth and the little people to be accommodated in any such plans. If the Master would have me go, I must. If he should have me stay, stay I must. In either eventualitye, I should not be content."

"Nay, Master Francis. Your dilemma was plain. But, 'tis my belief he left not these shores again; nor even attended a farther meeting of the Club."

"You have it already, sir; so that there is no excuse for my continuing to rattle upon't, but that to speak of him is like to his being alive; and there are few to whom I have opportunity to speak of him as I have to you."

"You honour me, in that respect, and I'm sensible of it. Here's the hare come. Take some more claret, good Francis, and let's hack on!"

"Your servant, sir!" He smiled and held forth his goblet in salute. "It came out that the Master's view of the affair was swiftley coming to resemble my own; so that, when the letter came next from the Chancellor to say that the request was denyd, he was not much dis-appointed.

"The journey was not render'd impossible, for the Exchequer was prepared that he should take a mortgage upon his pension; but the outcome of this would have been indebtedness at the end, which he would not permit, for he was desireous of compleating his plan in my regard.

"Then came time for Mister Boswell to return to Scotchland; so he, the Master and Sir Joshua shared a private dinner at Leicester Fields; and, after-ward, deliver'd Doctor Johnson at the entrance to Bolt-Court.

"The Doctor ask'd if Mister Boswell would come into the house, but he declin'd, for he had no wish to protract the parting; whereat the Doctor, who was then neither hale, nor sprightly, fair *trotted* away to where I awaited him in the court.

"The hackney-coach bore Mister Boswell out into the tumultuation of Fleet Street, and they never saw each other more."

"Do you believe that Johnson knew it was to be their last meeting?"

"Mister Boswell ask'd me the self-same question, sir; and, though I must own to being convinced for my own part, I cannot say with absolute certitude, either to him or to you, that it was the case,

"He did not come out and say that they should never meet again; nor did he make any other specifick reference to't. Conversely, he gave no positive impression that he anticipated such a meeting, for all that a certain correspondence past between them concerning a notion of Mister Boswell's to remouve to London. It never occur'd; and if 'twas referr'd to, the Doctor's invaryable response was: 'Poh! Poh!' and a change of topick."

"'Twas a sad occasion, then, Master Francis; the end of something unique and significant. 'Twere pity it shouldn't have lasted a bit longer."

"Others have exprest that view, sir, though I must say that I do not concur with it.

"Your inter-view with myself shall be compleat ere this day is done. You will have gain'd such impressions as you might, recorded such conversation as is of use, and you will do with it thereafter what you will.

"We have given to each other one day; and we have costed each other one day. If little or naught is gain'd; little or naught has been lost; and 'tis mete that it should be so.

"If you are desireous of recording my life, you have no obligation to constitute a major part of it your-self.

"Boswell admired the Master greatly, and the Master, in his turn, was passing fond of him; but, in Boswell's presence, the Master was ever a *specimen*.

"When he was on form, and giving forth of his wit and his knowledge, and taking all ways the advantage, 'twas fitting that he should have an admiring chronickler about him; 'twas e'en acceptable that the chronickler should propose topicks and other-wise stimulate the process.

"I must own to you that I can see little merit in his perpetual presence, when much mundane information may be drawn from those with more reason to be in attendaunce; and that I am well-pleas'd that Mister Boswell was elsewhere in periods of affliction, when still less would have been gain'd by his indelicate observation and chronickle-ising.

"No man is all performance, sir. Even Mister Garrick sometimes left the stage.

"Mister Boswell was Doctor Johnson's friend, I say, but he lov'd him as an exhibit. He has been a friend to me, also, and I say naught against his character, nor judge of him in any way, when I tell you that I deem'd it advantageous he should leave when he did."

"It seems we are apt to take certain things as granted. Those of my profession have a tendency to regard Boswell as the model in matters of biography. We are wont to assume that celebrated people court celebrity in all their doings. 'Tis certainly true that there are few aspects of a life such as Johnson's was that people do not wish to read about."

"That, I'll grant you; and do not think that I would invalidate Mister Boswell's performance as a writer of biography. He has been a most delicate selector of material.

"Still the selection was his, and not the Master's. What is there recorded is Mister Boswell's opinions and experiences in the Master's regard, with additional contributions. To produce such a work requires that the authour be present in as many circumstaunces as can be managd.

"You will have noted that the title of the performance is: 'Boswell's Life of Johnson', and not: 'Johnson's Life by Boswell'. Th'intent is clear enough, sir."

I had nothing to say to that; so sayd it.

"Now another trial was visited upon my Master. Mrs. Thrale decided to marry the Italian musician, Signor Piozzi."

"Ah. Now we are come to it! Why did her decision arouse so much ill-feeling?"

"There were varyous forms of ill-feeling involv'd, sir; not all proceeding from a common cause.

"The ill-feeling of Mrs. Thrale's off-spring took the form of jalousye, I believe. Like to most children, in my observation, the amourous fulfill-ment of their mother did not occupy a large portion of their concerns.

"Had she dy'd, and their father sought a replacement, they should have been equally oppos'd to't

"As it was, they had never exhibited any profound affection for Mister Henry, but would not easily see him replac'd – even had the pretender been English. 'Twas not so much *who* he was, as *that* he was, if you follow me.

"Until the matter is properly look'd at – and looking at the death of a parent is never attractive, sir – the assumption is that the widow'd shall remain true to the deceas'd beyond the grave. No logick in't; and that's the main reason for't.

"A parallel concern is the splitting of the family fortunes to accommodate the interloper. Indeed, there is ever the danger that the new object may receive a superior portion of both affection, and material demonstration thereof, than the fledg'd brood."

"Hah! That's true enough. But why was the *Doctor* so much against it?"

"That is a question, at once, more simple, and more complicated, sir.

"As I have sayd, the Master was particular-fond of young women, of which Mrs. Thrale was one; she being not a year or two either way of me, I should judge.

"She had marryed Mister Henry for his money and position (also, I believe, for her money; for it was conditional upon her making a match that had the approval of her benefactor!). They had not much to give, one to the other, in any other regard; save that he was sober and respectable, and she was decorous and respectable, likewise.

"He was very strict in his views, and his management of the house, denying his wyfe access to the kitchen, which he held to be his own preserve, and forbidding her the pleasures (which she believ'd them to be; and which I do not) of riding, bethinking the activity un-lady-like.

"She was much for the arts and stimulation, and would be involv'd in all that went forward. He was all dignity; a man for a-holding of his tongue and keeping his own counsel. They were in accord only in entertaining and travel, when his culinarye, and her interlocutory arts serv'd a common object.

"I'm certain that Doctor Johnson entertain'd great respect for Mister Henry. But he was also a little excessive in the employment of it. You may have read the account of how 'in command' of his wyfe Mister Thrale was, and wonder'd that the Doctor had not been mouv'd to record such assertions in, connexion with any other husband; not so, sir?"

The passage, from Boswell's *Life*, has Johnson as saying: 'I know no man who is more master of his wife and family than Thrale.' "I had not wonder'd at it, Master Francis. Nor am I convinced of the existence of any hidden significance in't now."

"In which, I am sure you are justify'd, sir. I would not have it other than that you should apply your discretion to all that I aver.

"I offer next his habitudinal appelation of her: *Mistress.*"

"This is naught but stuff, sir! Only a lunatick would call a woman 'mistress' in the presence of her husband, were she truly so. Let's have no more on't."

"Would not Mister Henry be expected to arrive at the same conclusion?"

"What? Enough, I say. This is calumny, upon your Master and benefactor. 'Tis not well done, and I'll have an end to't!"

"I must remind you, sir, that none knew my Master better than I; and none held – nay, still hold – him in higher esteem.

"A man is not made the greater by removing some of his parts. Indeed, be they his best parts or his worst, such a process cannot but *reduce* him.

"I have given an account of some of his afflictions, that you might see him in balaunce, as it should be. These afflictions were not just notes in a book, sir, but a plague which was about him for the whole of his life.

"Mister Boswell writes a categorye of thing here, another there; so we have a man of parts. When we speak of him, as when we speak of Williams, we make a reference to any particularityes of which the listener should be made aware.

"Mrs. Williams was blind. We use it as an explanation for the other matters we are to relate in her *connexion*. It is an aside which serves to identifye her for our reference.

"But, to Mrs. Williams, it was not an explanation, nor an aside, nor yet a reference

"If her blindness was incident to our perception of her, it was *essential* to her perception of all else. She did not cease to be blind when we refrain'd from thinking on't. She continued in that condition, even should she forget it herself.

"In description of her, we may clearly perceive the *effects* of her blindness; we may be shew'n with what success she triumph'd o'er it; and, if 'tis well done, we might come to know a deal *about* it. But we will not be shew'n the blindness its-self, sir; shall not see it; shall not know it.

"The labour of biography is to approximate, as closely as may be, what cannot be seen. All biography catalogues exterior show; more or less candidly, more or less percipiently, and more or less precisely.

"But, no matter how close to his subject the biographer should come, he cannot make the final move into that person's head; not, at least, by disinterested observation."

"Disinterest is the prime expedient of my profession."

"With respect, that is why your profession is bound to the mere observation of effect and consequence. Disinterest precludes imagination, which last is the only means by which kin-ship to real understanding may be achiev'd."

"But, a man may let his imagination get the better of him."

"So we must have discipline, and reason, and candour; but, just as we must have all of Johnson, so we must use *all* our means to capture him

"We may read Boswell's Johnson, first to last; or we may dip into him, here or there. We may take him from the shelf in an idle moment; or we may put him away for years together.

"If we would, truly, understand Johnson, we must first *read* Johnson. We are fortunate that we may do so; though many are content to read the biographer and the critick, taking no interest in the work.

"Then we may read biography and criticism; but, before we can draw a real picture therefrom, we must understand something of the biographer and the critick; for if we do not recognize their part, we cannot tell what parts belong to the subject; and, before we can embark upon this course, we must understand something of the possibilityes and limitations of biography.

"To Mister Boswell, Doctor Johnson was an admirable and estimable man.

"His biography is, therefore, the life of an admirable and estimable man, in which he does admirable and estimable things. If any one appear in the narrative to suggest un-admirable or in-estimable associations, they are shew'n to have done so from a want of admirability, estimability, or both, in them-selves.

"In short, Boswell provides an incomplete picture, as all biography must. But he has decided what picture he wishes to paint, and chosen his palette accordingly, throwing out the pigments he does not need.

"If a new light should subsequently fall upon the sitter, it does so to no effect, for Bozzy is without colours for its depiction.

"If you have read the Doctor's Life of Savage, you will find the same errour, for he, too, had a *motive*, to which his narrative is sub-servient; but you receive an advantage there, for Doctor Sam did not know Savage in his early life, and has merely copy'd another account; thus we have two men for the price of one – each irreconcileable with the other!"

"Still, master Francis! I retain a grip upon your coat-tails, but have had as much of fancy as I am dispos'd to take. Let's have your point, sir."

"Well, then, it is this, sir: biographyes and reports are precious powerful things, for they stand in the place of their subjects.

"If we consent to their alteration of those subjects, albeit on grounds of delicacy, we are party to mis-representation.

"Meeting the Doctor, in the flesh, as the saying is, so having a full-ish picture of him, Mister Boswell concludes that he is an admirable &c. By what right does he lay aside some of the evidence that brought him to that conclusion? Except, of course, that it is *his* life, and not the Doctor's.

"A true biography would offer every thing known or knowable about its subject, leaving the reader to discover cause for admiration or esteem. Johnson's Savage was two men; any real man may be a multitude. All his facets must be seen ere he can be truly valued.

"An *auto-biography* has more truth than a biography written by another, for it contains invariably something of the subject. Even if it be pack'd with lyes, they are the lyes of the subject; and, thus, of more assistaunce in his understanding than the flatterye of another."

"Is this the short version you are giving me?"

"That it is, sir," (laughing). "If we had the time, I could speak at some length upon the topick."

"Well, then, I thank you for your brevity!" We laugh'd heartily, and, taking up his goblet, he gave a toast.

"I give you *brevity*, sir. May there yet be time for a good deal more of it!

"Mister and Mrs. Thrale gave the Doctor the run of the house at Streatham, so that he even occasionally work'd upon his writing there: Mrs. T. acting amanuensis.

"The doing away with the formal introduction, which is ever attendant upon arrival and departure, left the mouvements of the varyous partyes un-accountable. Mister Thrale was usually at his business, or at the towne-house attached to the brewery at Deadman's Place, except at week-endings, when there was entertaining to be done.

"Mrs. Thrale was, therefore, very much in the company of the Doctor; they becoming firm friends, and he speaking to her as he spoke to no other woman that I knew of.

"His gyrations and his constant rocking to and fro' were consequent upon the pain with which he was cronickally rack'd. His first response to any discomfort was to put himself in motion,

"Apart from myself, I think only Mrs. Thrale was aware of this cause.

"Though he should use such motion as an expedient, he bethought himself, in the process, to be attempting to side-step the Lord's judgement; for that he was convinc'd that his afflictions were visited on him as a punishment for pleasure and indolence.

"Another aspect of his affliction concern'd dis-connexion. He had a terrour that, if he let his limbs cease to move, he might lose control of them, so that they might never move more.

"To ensure that feeling remain'd, he either continued in a state of motion, or resorted to inflicting pain upon himself.

"In some religious cultes, the practice of flagellation, and other forms of self-punishment is intrinsick. I believe there to be an element of this desire for corporeal exculpation in many who go to the Posture-Molls in Covent Garden. In any case, I'm certain that such a motive was present in the Master.

"I'll own that the suggestion does not sit easy, having about it a necessary connotation of degradation; but, we must keep in mind that degradation is part of the object of the punishment as ecclesiastically practised, and must surely remain so in its parodye."

"Is not such pious degradation intended solely for the attention of the Redeemer?"

"In its pure form, it surely hath redemption as its object, sir. My Burton's Book, Number twenty: 'History of the Lives of English Divines' details Thos. Becket's practise of donning an hair shirt in a spirit of self-degradation and exculpation.

"The reasoning of it seems to go: that there shall be no remaining necessity for the sinner to be subjected to ignominy, nor yet the fireye torments, hath he but caus'd his body to be used in a degraded fashion. A low reading of the All-mighty's moral intent, in my view, sir."

"Tarry there, Master Francis. Let's have no blasphemy. You may be quite right in what you say; but be steady – there are others present who might take exception." Although we were quite remouv'd from the main part of the saloon, 'twere wiser to remain upon the safer side, and give no cause for religious quarrelling.

"Point taken, sir. I am ever inclin'd to be carry'd off by my subject."

"There's naught against that."

"Nay, sir; but a man who runneth into the path of a carriage is apt to be mow'n down!"

"You have it exact, Master Francis. Running is sublime sport when the field is clear, but you had best be a little fancy with your feet when you get in the alleys."

"As you say, sir."

The jugg'd hare, and a fair quantity of bread and vegetables having been nicely dispatch'd, my thoughts turn'd to the plum-duff, which the house offer'd in dessert. I was not sure if 'twould be a prudent thing for my un-molar'd friend.

"What say you to plum-duff, Master Francis?"

"That I should take it above flagellation ev'ry time, sir!"

"Ha! Then we are of a mind on that account!" I call'd the serving-wench, bidding her produce some of the fine dessert for my companion and myself; which done, Master Francis went on.

"Returning, then, to the reasons for Doctor Johnson's objections to the marriage to Piozzi, I believe they were two-fold.

"Whether we find it to our taste, or not, one of those reasons had to do with being found out.

"I know that he and she had in their possession manacles, chains, and other related engines. The house, like any such, was full of whips. I cannot claim to have been present at the using of them; but neither can I, in all conscience, claim that they were ornamental in purpose.

"I know enough of the character, and of the concatenation of afflictions, of my Master, to know, likewise, that this form of diversion would afford him some satisfaction. Perhaps relief is more apposite.

"I have seen him apply pain to one part of his person, in order to obtain relief in another; a process I have tryd myself, with a measure of success, further emboldening my conviction.

"I only repeat, sir, that I never lov'd him any the less for't. Indeed, if we cease to pull pious faces, 'twas but another facet of his humanity. Each man must contrive to bear his cross in the manner he is fitted so to do.

"Had he been still youthfull and vigourous, he might have told all, and talk'd himself into the right; for he'd no taste for hypocrisy while he'd yet the strength to spit it out; but, being low of tone, he fear'd and doubted and held his tongue.

"He might also, as I dared to offer earlier in the day, have taken her to his own wyfe; for, manacles or not, there was a deep and genuine affection between them. They were much in the same mould for both witty talk and the taking of offense. He was inordinately fond of her children; and, if they must suffer paternal substitution, they would suffer it from him before many.

"Albeit there was not much left of his life to give to her, and nursing should predominate in such as there was, but the measure of happiness for all concern'd would have been much the greater.

"None, were they children, neighbours, visitors, or biographers, should have snubb'd either Thrale or Johnson; and they should not have shunn'd each other."

"Believe you that Johnson was, himself, aware of this?"

"Yes, sir; but not until the marriage to Signor Piozzi was already in hand. He had, without a doubt, had it in his mind to take another wyfe, after the death of Mrs. Johnson, the first; but he lack'd confidence with the kind of women he really lov'd. He believ'd himself riddl'd with defects, and was sure that no woman who was not wanting in some fashion herself would be doing with such a man as he, lest it be for some more nefarious motive, for he could not conceive of his love being truly reciprocated.

"There, then, are his reasons for criticising, and taking against Mrs Thrale: shame and guilt. He was ashamed of the goings on while Mister Henry yet liv'd; and he was guilty that he did not bring himself to propose matrimony in the Italian's place.

"Which brings us, at last, to Mrs. Thrale's reasons for claiming that her entire relationship with the Doctor had been a burthen plac'd upon her, which she had supported in duty to her late husband.

"If. you read her earlier eulogyes and panegyricks upon this man, whom she now profess'd to have ever regarded with disgust, you may dismiss it as nonsense forthwith.

"When Mister Henry dy'd, he left her comfortable; but he left her young, and he left her lonely, sir.

"'Twas not reasonable that she should live out a quiet life in that grand house, after the companye she had kept. She had known Signor Piozzi previous, and he took up the running, as the saying is. If the Doctor had advanced himself, I think she'd have had him. I think she even expected that he should make overtures.

"But, he did not; and, worse from her side, he did not support her choice.

"She believ'd that he respected her, not just for her hostessing and her prittiness, but for her wit, and her intelligence. When he seem'd to go agin her, she took it amiss, on the ground that he did not grant her enough sense to choose whom she should marry.

"The truth of it was other, of course. He was agin it, for he wanted her himself; but was ill-humour'd because he'd done nothing about it.

"As I sayd, she was well-school'd at the taking of offense, and did so in dramatick fashion. But she also felt shame now about the doings with the chains, which made her still more tetchy, and prone to find fault with the Master.

"Finally, having embark'd upon a course, she, like the Master, was not easy to bring about. Having abus'd him, then, 'twere nigh impossible that she should retract. She must, in stead, shew herself to have been right by giving out more of the same; which is what she did, sir.

"If the Doctor had not been so intransigent, she might have given a little, and a reconciliation: manag'd.

"But, in truth, no one behaved well in the entire affair, and we'd as well blame the positions of the stars and have done with it.

"The Doctor dy'd with the thing un-resolv'd; and he was the only one who could have alter'd her mind.

"In her heart, and in her private chamber, she knows the truth of it; but the truth (whether it be as I surmise it, or some other) will likely dye when she does; and, when that time comes, we shall be left only with books – Boswell's, hers, the Knight's, &c.

"There's no altering *their* minds, sir."

CHAPTER SIXTEEN

IN WHICH WE LEARN OF DOCTOR JOHNSON'S LAST DAYS

The repast done with, we elected to finish our time together as it had begun, with some more of Lichfield's famous ale. The evening was drawing on, and I began to fear for the time that we must call a halt to our converse, so determin'd was I that the full measure should be had from what had, at first, seem'd little more than an idle proposition.

We took our ease now, that digestion of the hare and the plums might be facilitated, and I bade Master Barber take up his narrative.

"In the middle of that final year, while the climate was for it, the Doctor set about a-putting of his affairs in order.

"He first wrote to the Reverend Mister Bagshaw at Bromley Church, sending him an inscription to be put upon Mrs. Johnson's grave. He had already discuss'd this with Mister Ryland, the West Indian merchant, on Tower Hill, who would take in charge the supply and the carving of a stone for the purpose.

"On the day following, we departed for Lichfield and Ashbourne; a visit to these places which would be my first, and his last.

"It took us two days to come here, and we remain'd for five, but the Doctor now found walking nigh impossible, so was not able to go abroad much. His asthma troubled him greatly, and the opium that he had been used to take when the fits were upon him, though it gave him sufficient of relief that he might sleep or lye tranquille, no longer discover'd strength enough in him for perambulation.

"At the conclusion of the five days, therefore, we mov'd on from Miss Porter's Bread-Court to the Reverend Doctor Taylor's at Ashbourne in Derbyshire.

"There, the Doctor began to shew some improuv'ment; being able, after a short while, to go to church, and also to visit the stately house of the Duke and Duchess of Devonshire at

Chatsworth; which was a place of marvells without end, sir; such water-falls and feats of construction have been wrought in the gardens there, as defy belief. Also, they have an huge household, though I was upon mine honour to Elizabeth, and spent such time as I had in reading.

"Even the Doctor's dropsy abated a second time, so that he was much more himself when such as Mister Windham came to call upon him at Ashbourne.

"But he had now come to that which he abhorr'd in others, in that he was much exercis'd by the weather."

"It cannot be denyd to be a matter of the greatest moment to us all, Master Francis. Be we humble or great, we are ever subject to its humeurs. As you have so ably inferr'd with respect to other, and un-connected, matters, we shall never master the climate by the process of ignoring it."

"Think you that we shall someday master it, sir?"

"Not in a sense of controlling its behaviour, Master Francis; but 'tis certainly my view that we shall much improuve our skill in its prediction, so that we might navigate our passage through't the better."

"There's another interesting parallel there then, sir; for a servant, of a man or of a government, will not come to a position of control, neither; but may be strikingly effectual and successful in his own purpose, if he can but accurately identifye the mind, and predict the behaviour of, those he must call master."

"I like it well, Master Francis; well, indeed. Meteorology is, then, the science of life its-self!" We laugh'd much at this.

"You are at liberty to draw that conclusion, sir. 'Tis surely as good as any presently in existence!"

"What would our Johnson have made of that, would you think?"

My companion clapt one hand to his chest, and drew him-self to his full height (no great distance). Then, in a measured tone, with a slight hint of Staffordshire, he announc'd: "Sir, a man who is tired of London, is tired of fore-casting the weather!"

He was much restor'd now, having cast off completely the

low-spirits with which he had been smitten upon our earlier
visit to his house in Stow-street. He appear'd to be a man made
for companye and entertainment, though having much of the
serious philosopher about him. His thoughts, and his humour
were both such as would be an asset at most tables. Only a want
of prudence in manner and speech (ally'd to his subterranean
birth and station) should make of him a *pariah*, as the Indians
have it.

"You think passing well, Master Francis. Have you
contemplated following your Master's steps and becoming an
authour?"

"Contemplated, yes, sir; but I have not the persistence for't,
and I doubt if I should obtain a single sub-scription."

"I understand your fellow-African, – he that you mention'd
in connexion with his grosserye shop – Mister Ignatius Sancho,
has some success in that form of endeavour."

"His case and mine are not identical, though we be both
call'd African, sir. He moves much in polite and decorous
circles – if not in person, in the form of his musick, which is
most popular in the with-drawing rooms of London and Bath, I
believe.

"Apart from his association with Mister Sterne, he has his
musick as evidaunce that there is something about him."

"Do you not write, though, from the pure motive of
recording your philosophy?"

"No, sir. The master of my education taught me that none
but a blockhead writes, except for money; and my writing
should bring me naught of that.

"That consideration aside, I have oft thought that a good
purpose would be serv'd by my writing my life-story; but I
knew not where to begin, so began not at all – and now I have
you to do it for me!"

"Hah! Your servant, sir."

Master Barber return'd again to the last months of Johnson's
life. "We continued at Ashbourne until the August, at which
time the Doctor felt better able to benefit from re-visiting
Lichfield.

"Accordingly, we set out in Doctor Taylor's personal coach (a fine contraption, sir, with two livery'd postillions in the best style), to be deliver'd again to Miss Lucy's house.

"Whilst there, an exchange took place which, incidentally, re-enforced some of the things I have said about his forebearaunce and his attitude to life, with its attendant pains.

"Miss Seward came to call upon him frequently in the course of our sojourn, on one occasion imparting a story concerning a learned pig – a pig, this was, which had been school'd in divers activityes more the province of horses and dogs.

"The Doctor was ever taken with such singular particulars, and rais'd considerably in humour in the course of their relating.

"At the conclusion of Miss S-'s account, he said: 'Then the pigs are a race un-justly calumniated. *Pig* has, it seems, not been wanting to *man,* but *man* to *pig.* We do not allow *time* for his education, we kill him at a year old.'

"The Reverend Mister White, who was also present, said that 'great torture must have been employ'd ere the indocility of the animal could have been subdued.'

"'Certainly', replyd the Doctor, turning back to Miss Seward, 'but, how old is your pig?' Miss Seward told him that the pig was three years old, at which he concluded: 'The pig has no cause to complain; he would have been kill'd the first year if he had not been educated, and protracted existence is a good recompense for very considerable degrees of torture.'."

"I must own that his statement does seem to support your premise, Master Francis. Was not the case of the pig singular?"

"'Tis my view that we habitually under-value the intelligence of our fellow-creatures, sir.

"Our interest lies elsewhere; just as a Frenchie can look at an horse, which we regard as an animal of some intelligence, and see only meat, we also develop ways of looking at God's creatures that suit our purpose.

"We tell our-selves that fish are incapable of any feeling, and angling becomes an innocent pursuit. Yet, if fish felt naught, they would have no reason to resist our poor attempts at their capture.

"Look upon a fish as it violently thrashes upon the bank, vainly attempting to catch its watery breath, and tell me it feels naught."

"But men of science have prov'd it, my friend."

"*Admirable Curiosityes of Nature & Art*, sir; that is the *Burton's* book in question. A glorify'd fish-monger, having minutely examin'd of his fillets, has found no nerves of the required sort. Proof of naught except of its-self, sir!

"I say to men of science, sir: if you would know aught of living fishes, observe living fishes; for if once a fish is dead, it is just that.

"A live hare is an animal of intelligence and feeling; a jugg'd hare is a supper – since the eating of which, I have wander'd too often from the topick we are here to discuss.

"The Doctor was in no doubt about the proximity of his death. As I said previous, he was about the business of getting his affairs in order.

"It might have been imagin'd that he would choose to end his days where they began, here in Lichfield; for here were many as cared for him greatly, and there were none of the in-mates waiting, for him in London.

"It should have been the most poetickal finish, but he still had matters to conclude; and I believe that it was in his nature to be at the centre of the life he had him-self created, rather than at the point of his own creation; in which he may have been right.

"He had friends of long-standing at Birmingham, so 'twas there that we went next, staying a few days, before moving, for the last time, to Oxford.

"This place had play'd a large part in the Master's life, since leaving Lichfield to make his fortune in the Capital; so it was fitting, perhaps, that it should have been the locus of his last visit; the object of his ultimate jaunt.

"He told Doctor Adams that he was now well enough, and of a consentaneous frame of mind to embark upon the prayer-book mooted upon our previous visit.

This would be his 'Prayers and Meditations', which he

deliver'd to the Reverend Mister Strahan, son of the printer.

"After about a week, we return'd to London, arriving in about the middle of November, as I recall.

"He had never really allow'd a co-relation between health and climate, as we have seen; but, I fear he was mis-taken not to see it; for, at Ashbourne, where there is purity and freshness; where the aire is clear and the water likewise, his asthma fell from him, and his dropsy flow'd away.

"While he was here in Lichfield, 'twas the same. Having had the time to recover, he stayed recovered in this idyllick place.

"Naught much at Birmingham to do him harm, neither; and Oxford, too, is about as far remov'd as you can get from the commotion and squalour of his adopted home.

"Hardly had he arriv'd back in that place, than both afflictions made a new appearaunce.

"I fear I cannot wonder at it, when I look back upon it from here.

"Mid-winter in London is not a thing to be easily borne, e'en by those with youth and health to aid them.

"Cold aires and draughts are everywhere, the alleys and wynds providing means for their acceleration, the courts and yards preventing their passing. Vapours from the stinking ditches rise, to be met with the black smoak of the many thousand fyres, so that they commingle together, and hang upon the aire, where they may be joyn'd by the fetid stench of the charnel houses, the noxious tallow from the chandlers, and those things beyond description that are carry'd upon the river.

"Everywhere is filth and dust, so that every man seems to carry the dis-ease of hundreds, in his nostrils, on his boots, and upon the brim of his hat.

"No wonder, I say, that a man already low, should be broken in such a place.

"When he is not beset with the stuff of plague and vapour, he must look upon the most shocking and dis-heartening things to be seen in the kingdom: the de-form'd, the pox-ridden, the consumptives, the starvelings; the children of the whores for sale at Charing Cross; the heads of the executed upon the gates.

"Is that a centre of a civilization, sir?"

"The displaying of the heads, at least, is no more, Master Francis."

"Well, then, that is something; but a great deal more must find alteration in that pestilent place ere I should find reason to go there more.

"Nay, sir; I'm a *Lichfield* man!"

"Ha! I trust the place shall be as generous in *your* adoption, good Francis!"

We crash'd our tankards together in the manner of workmen. "Lichfield," we cry'd in unison.

"My Master's preparations for the end went forward in earnest now, for he knew with a certainty that it was high.

"He had Mister Green, the apothecary here, attend to the placing of an engrav'd stone flag in the aisle of St. Michael's Church, In Memoriam of his brother, mother and father.

"That done, he mov'd on to death quite rapidly.

"Many of his friends and admirers came to Bolt-Court to pay homage to him, and to bring such comfort as they might. Doctors came and went, and some particular friends were almost constantly about him.

"Some of the doctors held him in such high regard that they demanded no fees for their ministrations, sir; which included Heberden and Brocklesby, aforemention'd.

"John De Mullin was of great assistaunce to me at this time; for it fell to me to carry out the instructions of the doctors during the hours of darkness, and it was a fair burden for one, sir. Especially that I became very sentimental, when alone, and found it hard to be as strong as the Doctor needed me to be.

"John's presence gave me that extra strength, both physically and spiritually, so that I was not so grief-stricken; and also had another pair of hands to assist in the Master's lifting and moving. He needed sitting up, or turning at constant intervals, throughout the day and night, sir, as you might imagine; to guard against the choaking and the sores. His legs had become horrible bloated with the waters of the dropsy, giving him great pain, and making it impossible for him to move anywhere of his own volition – although he, several times, insisted that he be lifted to the floor, where he could adopt a praying position.

"Sometimes, I thought his agony should be the end of me, I was so solicitous of his health, sir. I often return'd to Elizabeth, when John gave me leave, and just wept until I was a-sleep.

"Then, one night, when John and myself were together in the chamber, we were aware of the Master doing something under the cover; which pulling back, we discover'd that he had laid hold of one of the doctors' lancets, and meant to pierce his legs with it, in the cause of evacuation of the waters.

"Fearing far worse consequences, John and I fell upon him, and try'd to wrest the lancet from his hand; in which we succeeded at last; the Master crying: 'Scoundrel' at me, and threatening to stab Master John.

"We were most shook by this, as you might have suspected; both by the incident, and by the abuse we receiv'd for our faithfull-ness to the Master.

"We went aside, for the briefest possible of interludes, while we be-calm'd each other and agreed that 'twas only the Doctor's extremity as had call'd him to behave contrary to his character; when he gave a loud cry, and we ran to his bed-side.

"Pulling down the cover a second time, we discover'd that he had gone forward with his plan, regardless of our pre-caution, with a pair of scissors from the bed-side chest.

"There are not sufficient terms in my vocabulary to describe to you the horrour John and I experience'd at that time, sir. Anything that would perform the office of a rag was brought so that we might staunch the flow, as we thought it, of the Master's vital fluids.

"Realizing now the inevitability of the situation, he demanded that Doctor Brocklesby tell him plain if there were any hope of recovery.

"That good and brave man made no pretense, but told him what he knew in his heart.

"I need not tell you, for all that, that we kept him constantly in our sight from that night forward. Indeed, I could hardly bear to be parted from him at all, fearing that he should attempt something of that sort again.

"But, as the end approach'd, more people came about him, and I was able to sleep a little now and again.

"When he was come to, he was much concern'd with his spiritual preparation, and had me pray with him. 'Attend, Francis, to the salvation of your soul, which is the object of greatest importance,' he told me, though I did not immediately comprehend the truth of what he said.

"On his last day, Miss Morris, the child of a close friend, came to the street-door, and asked that she might receive the Doctor's blessing. It was an odd thing, or it seem'd so at the time. But the whole world seem'd strange, as if time had stopt, and there was no noise carrying into the court from Fleet Street. There seem'd even to be no smell upon the aire.

"I went to see if the Master was able to receive her, but found she had follow'd me into the chamber.

"'Miss Morris earnestly desires of you that you might consent to give her your blessing, Master Sam,' says I; at which, he manag'd to turn himself in the bed:

"'God bless you, my dear!'

"I shew'd the girl out and return'd to the chamber, where Mrs. De Mullin was; and we sat together, in silence, while the Master's asthmatick beathing became ever louder. There was naught we could do now, but wait.

"Then, around seven o'clock in the evening, the breathing stopt. I walk'd slowly over to him and checked for signs of life as the doctors had shewn me how; but he was no more.

"I shouted his name after him, with all the strength I could find, and fell, exhausted, upon his empty body."

CHAPTER SEVENTEEN

IN WHICH OUR INTERVIEW REACHES ITS CONCLUSION AND MASTER BARBER EXPOSES THE NATURE AND FULL EXTENT OF HIS TROUBLESOME DISORDER

Doctor Samuel Johnson died upon Monday, the thirteenth day of December, One-Thousand-Seven-Hundred-and-Eighty-Four, and was buryed at Westminster Abbey, a week later.

"So it was ended, Master Francis."

"Aye, sir; it was ended. Pain was ended. Un-certainty was ended. Wit was ended. Writing was ended. Gyrating was ended.

"Beyond all, sir, the life was ended."

"The Life of Johnson was ended 'tis true; but, to employ your own devyse, was not your next life beginning?"

"Oh, yes, sir; that it was, and I less prepar'd for it than the last."

"Surely you knew he must die."

"I knew it very well, sir; but, while he liv'd, I thought only of him. I had not contemplated what effect his passing would have upon myself.

"As I have told you, my life contain'd but two certaintyes; two things upon which I could rely, what-ever else might try my reason.

"One was the persistence of the Master himself; the other, my vow to serve him.

"We have discuss'd how the Johnson that exists in Boswell's book has been granted his existence by Boswell. That is to say that he is not the real Johnson; he who died at Bolt-Court; but a Johnson of Boswell's fancy.

"There is another Johnson of Mrs Piozzi's fancy; and still another of the Knight's.

"None is the genuine Johnson, but together they contain much of him; and, at least, they had the real one as their subject.

"Since he was an authour, we are fortunate too, in that we have his own words to know him by.

"My Master had a real existence in many people's minds, and shall persist in counterfeit form, for as long as there are books.

"But my case is different, sir, for I have produc'd no books, and I have been the subject of no books, nor even of prosopography (until today).

"I, sir, am oppress'd with a troublesome disorder, which I have only lately come to apprehend.

"None of my lives has had independent purpose, sir. If there be none other to serve, my living is without point."

"That cannot be."

"But, it is, sir. Why did you take the trouble to seek me out? Not for myself, but because I was Doctor Johnson's faithfull servant."

"I'll grant you that was my original purpose, but you would be unjust to suggest it is the reason for my remaining in your company thus long."

"Nay, sir; 'twas not a slur; merely an illustration.

"I have been in *life* what the Doctor became in *death*: a man with no existence, except as an adjunct to another.

"Only in my sea-life was I sufficient in myself; and recorded as such. In my Johnsonian life, I am only a 'Frank was there', 'Make the coffee, Frank', or 'Frank came behind'."

"Is this not self-pity, Master Francis? There are others who are less chronicl'd even than you: Poll, Betsy – even Elizabeth."

"I won't deny the truth in that, sir; but it is not *chronicklinq* that concerns me. I am *chronickl'd* passing well, in truth, for I make a proportionate appearance to the degree of my achievement."

"Nay, Francis, you wrong yourself by saying so. You were of much comfort and assistaunce to your Master, and did a great deal of which we can be aware, though it be not recorded. He was fortunate indeed to be the recipient of your devotion at the end, and in other periods of in-disposition."

"I thank you for saying so, sir. I have acquir'd the habit of self-censure, which few men have try'd to deter me from. But chronickles be still chronickles, sir; and a life is a life.

"When the Doctor died, I had a life given to me, I had

property given to me, and I had money given to me; but I had no use for any of them."

"You had a beautiful wyfe, and children; and you are an intelligent and able man. They should have been a godsend to you."

"But that is the nature of my disorder, sir. I could make nothing of any of these things.

"To a slave, a dream of running away is sufficient to keep something of the spirit alive. Most slaves never do it, but their dream of it helps them bear with their captivity. The word 'freedom' to a slave means 'running away'. He has absolutely no idea what he will do when he runs away; the running away is an end unto itself; because ideas of what to do are of no use to a slave.

"If your life belongs to another, there's nothing to be gain'd from making plans for the future. It is not your future to plan; so you go from day to day, and the only dream you allow yourself is that, one day, you will run away.

"When I came into Doctor Johnson's house-hold, it matter'd not how benevolent were his intentions for the rest of my life. I had a chance to run away, and I took it. I should have done so, even if Colonel Bathurst had not 'given' me my freedom; but, since he did, I felt still more justify'd in doing it.

"Only in doing it does the slave come to the realization that it is not the panacea he has all-ways believ'd it to be. Unless you go on running, you must arrive at something. But you cannot tell when you have arriv'd, because you have no place in mind.

"A free man knows what he would have from life; what he would do to achieve it. A freed man knows but one life; that from which he has escap'd or been releas'd. He is only clear upon what he doesn't want; what he won't do.

"It is a hard lesson to learn that you are not fitted to live your own life, sir. I learnt it when I ran away the first time from Gough Square. That's why I went to the Navy, the second time. In the service of the King, a man may be a man, yet still have no responsibility.

"I did not run away from the Navy, sir. The joining of it had been my choice.

"For the first time in my life, I had made a decision, not just to run from something, but to choose somewhere to run to. This may seem a trifle to a free-born Englishman, but it was progress of some magnitude to me, sir."

"Not at all. I understand you very well. Far from regarding it as a trifle, I am more than sensible of what a proof it is of superior intellect on your part, to have recognis'd such shortcomings in yourself. 'Tis not a common ability, Francis, you may be sure."

"Well then, sir, you might also appreciate how unwelcome was the Doctor's intercession for my dis-charge."

"You said earlier that you were content in your sea-life."

"Aye, but 'twas more than that, sir. A-joining of the Navy was the single positive thing I had done in my life, which was entirely of mine own origination. It was, in short, the only life which was mine. But I was not to be allow'd it.

"I bethought myself free as the wind; out of reach, upon the sea; but all was delusion.

"The Doctor's benignant slavery could lay hold upon me even at so great a distance."

"How can you call your Master's treatment of you slavery?"

"Bah, sir 'Tis true that he used no manacles or chains (he'd other uses for them), but he tether'd me just as fast.

"A landman in His Majesty's Service may receive a letter. He sent me none. A free man may give an opinion as to whether he would go ashore or remain at sea. He never ask'd for anything of that sort.

"Regardless of my feelings, he interceded with the powerfull, because he wanted me to return to his companye.

"Were that not slavery, sir?"

"I'm un-easy about the terminology, Francis. I have found our meeting and discussions most congenial, and have come to like you very well. Much of what you have advanc'd has caus'd me to alter my thinking, but I must own to finding the present proposition un-gracious, to say the least."

"Gracious-ness is seldom the shortest path to truth, sir."

"He gave you such freedom; he had you educated; and he left you money and propertye."

"Aye, sir. Many were the things he did, on my behalf; many the decisions taken; many the improvements made. Benignant slavery, I say again, sir.

"I was no more fitted to direct my own life upon leaving his service, than I was when I first came to him. In thirty-five years, I'd had no practise at it.

"The Knight fear'd that we would have too much of luxury after the Doctor's death, and he was right. We have had the luxury of abuse from those who would not have deigned to speak to us before; we've had the luxury of being surrounded by possessions we must be careful of, because every one still thinks of them as the Doctor's; and we've had the luxury of ill-ness, which we could no-wise afford before the legacy.

"Everything I have told you today is true, sir; including that I lov'd my master, and that he lov'd me; but it was as man and favourite dog.

"You ask'd earlier why we remov'd to Lichfield following his death. 'Twas to complete the circle of his influence, sir; to return to the point of creation, so that I might take hold of my own life, while some of it is left to me.

"His money is now almost gone, so that I can see the possibility of forming my own actions again."

I could find nothing to say to Master Barber. I had been open to his curious philosophy, and had found much in it, but I felt nothing would be serv'd by continuing in this vein. The image of his wyfe floated back into my mind, standing in the red-glow upon the step of the house in Stow-street: "I'm sure that you will employ your highest judgement and discretion in recording what passes between you.

"Our lives have seen us high and low by turns, and we expect no alteration to the pattern hereafter. Our connexions to the wise have given us enough of wisdom to fulfil our destiny, and to pass on such as we have to others.

"If some record of our being goes forward, it is all that we can ask."

GENTLEMAN' S MAGAZINE February 1801

OBITUARY

Died on the 13th. February at the Infirmary at Stafford, where he was under the care of the surgeons of that useful institution for a painful operation,

MR. FRANCIS BARBER,

the faithful servant and residuary legatee of Dr. Samuel Johnson, of whose life since the death of his much-loved Master, we shall be glad to receive particulars.

Mr. Barber was a married man, and gave to his wife, enamelled for a mourning ring, the wedding ring which his Master had carefully preserved as a memorial of his *Tetty*

GENTLEMAN' S MAGAZINE February 1818

MINOR CORRESPONDENCE

Mr. Thomas Simpson, Esq., says:

Perhaps it may not be generally known that there is now in the possession of a gentleman, who purchased it of Mrs. Barber, the wife of Francis Barber, Dr. Johnson's faithful servant, the original miniature, painted about the year 1736, of the late Dr. Samuel Johnson, when he was in his twenty-eighth year.

It is in good preservation, and is the only one ever painted at so early a period of his life.

It was given by the Doctor himself to Mrs. Barber, who died at Lichfield about two years since, a short time before his death, with an injunction that she should never make it known; which request was strictly complied with until her poverty obliged her to dispose of it to its present possessor

Printed in the United Kingdom
by Lightning Source UK Ltd.
125703UK00001B/334-354/A